HEALTHCARE MARKETING

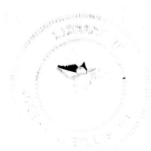

HEALTHCARE MARKETING

A CASE STUDY APPROACH

Leigh W. Cellucci · Carla Wiggins · Tracy J. Farnsworth

AUPHA

Health Administration Press, Chicago, Illinois
AUPHA Press, Arlington, Virginia

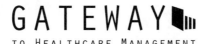

TO HEALTHCARE MANAGEMENT

Library of Congress Cataloging-in-Publication Data

Cellucci, Leigh W.
  Healthcare marketing : a case study approach / Leigh W. Cellucci, Carla Wiggins, and Tracy J. Farnsworth.
      pages cm
  Includes index.
  ISBN 978-1-56793-605-6 (alk. paper)
  1. Medical care--Marketing--Case studies. 2. Health services administration--Case studies. I. Wiggins, Carla.
II. Farnsworth, Tracy J. III. Title.
  RA410.56.C45 2014
  362.1068'8--dc23
                          2013027147

The paper used in this publication meets the minimum requirements of American National Standard for Information Sciences—Permanence of Paper for Printed Library Materials, ANSI Z39.48-1984.♾™

Acquisitions editor: Carrie McDonald and Janet Davis; Project manager: Jennifer Seibert; Cover designer: Marisa Jackson; Layout: Cepheus Edmondson

Found an error or typo? We want to know! Please email it to hapbooks@ache.org, and put "Book Error" in the subject line.

For photocopying and copyright information, please contact Copyright Clearance Center at www.copyright
.com or (978) 750-8400.

Health Administration Press
A division of the Foundation
   of the American College of
   Healthcare Executives
One North Franklin Street,
Suite 1700
Chicago, IL 60606-3529
(312) 424-2800

Association of University Programs
   in Health Administration
2000 North 14th Street
Suite 780
Arlington, VA 22201
(703) 894-0940

BRIEF CONTENTS

DETAILED CONTENTS

FOREWORD

As financial pressures on healthcare delivery organizations continue to tighten, every dollar devoted to marketing comes under scrutiny. As one of a dwindling number of discretionary expenditures in a budget, the marketing line looks ripe for cutting. People inside and outside the organization wonder what the marketing department does and why it should receive funding.

In *Healthcare Marketing: A Case Study Approach*, Leigh Cellucci, Carla Wiggins, and Tracy Farnsworth answer these questions with cogent descriptions of the activities healthcare marketing professionals engage in every day. They weave these descriptions into a compelling text that will help aspiring marketing staffers better understand their role and put into perspective the challenges they face in modern healthcare delivery organizations.

The strength of this book rests on a set of highly realistic cases prepared by the authors. In my 26 years of business experience, I have encountered exactly the same kinds of situations and problems depicted in this book, and the authors' ability to frame these problems in their text will help readers understand the many pressures on marketing staffers as well as on the executives who oversee their activities. Each chapter begins with a case study that sets the stage for key decisions marketers and their supervisors need to make, and the authors do an excellent job of drawing attention to the organization's mission, vision, and values as a lens through which to interpret problems and develop solutions.

The authors also help fill a void in readers' understanding by focusing on smaller markets and rural health systems, which are often overlooked in healthcare management texts and where marketers experience different kinds of challenges and serve unique population segments. As the executives of these organizations work to meet the needs of their markets, they lack the scale—and the resources—of major market hospitals, medical practices, and media partners. They have to rely on their wits and creativity, and the authors do an excellent job of portraying the special conditions faced by marketing staff working in this environment.

The authors' message is timely and important: Marketing in healthcare continues to evolve, and the job of the contemporary marketing professional will constantly change. This book sheds new light on this essential work.

John W. Huppertz, PhD
Union Graduate College
Schenectady, New York

PREFACE

In the fall of 2008, the Association of University Programs in Health Administration (AUPHA) held its biennial undergraduate workshop in Nashville, Tennessee. Professors were provided opportunities to network, visit with one another, and discuss what they needed to make their courses better. One theme that emerged from the discussions among professors in health administration programs was the need for healthcare marketing texts that fit their courses and their students. The conversations held at that meeting motivated us to write this book.

Specifically, the healthcare marketing conversations centered on a simple, shared theme: Business-focused marketing themes *sometimes* fit healthcare marketing efforts. We all need to know who our target market is, for example. However, when we engaged our healthcare marketing students in community projects (e.g., assisting with the preparation of a marketing plan for a local community healthcare center, helping to design a press release regarding the acquisition of the da Vinci robot at a regional medical center), we were introducing them to projects that were like business marketing yet different. We realized our need to embrace the fact that the healthcare industry is unique and thus so are its marketing needs.

We created this textbook to focus on the uniqueness of marketing in the healthcare industry, applying general marketing theory and concepts where appropriate and including real case examples of healthcare marketing professionals' experiences. Healthcare professionals understand that healthcare marketing is not general marketing in a different industry that just happens to be healthcare. As one healthcare marketer from a for-profit hospital stated during a December 2010 interview:

> The 4 Ps in marketing—price, place, promotion, and product? They don't fit for us. We [the hospital] are not about price. We do not control price, except perhaps for cosmetic surgeries; place—our hospital is where it is. Need surgery? You come to us, if the physician refers you. We think about the 4 Ps in healthcare marketing as patients, physicians, public, and payers. Healthcare marketing is different than regular marketing, and my people know that.

Additionally, the success of the Gateway series by Health Administration Press attests to a true need for health administration textbooks written for undergraduate students and programs as well as for entry-level personnel in hospitals, clinics, healthcare centers, and physician practices.

Moreover, we wanted to create a text that would engage students in the activities and work they will be involved in and responsible for when they become healthcare marketing professionals. To that end, we blend theory and practical applications to keep students interested and the topics relevant. The applied learning experiences in this text, based on real-life healthcare marketing events, are presented in three formats:

1. **Case studies** presented at the beginning of each chapter introduce students to the themes of the discussion that follows.

2. **Exercises** presented at the end of each chapter have students apply concepts they have learned to real-life healthcare marketing situations.

3. **Feature cases** presented at the beginning of each part of the book engage students in an in-depth analysis of issues discussed in the ensuing chapters.

The feature cases are substantial and reflect real-life situations. Some modifications to names, case settings, and numerical values have been made to preserve anonymity and accentuate points of learning. The first case, "Hospital Consolidation," invites students to consider the dynamic relationship healthcare providers have with their local and regional market and to appreciate the need to balance the interests of the organization and the community when making important decisions that affect the healthcare marketplace. In this case, the participants' and facilities' names and various numerical values have been changed.

The second case, "Market Management," challenges students to analyze and prioritize various kinds of information common to a dynamic and competitive healthcare marketplace for use in an organization's strategic marketing process. Information from this case is derived from *California Health Care Almanac*, a publication of the California Health-Care Foundation. Although the information related to the Fresno, California, healthcare market is unchanged, the characters, including their roles and actions, are fictitious.

The third case, "Palomar Heart Hospital," helps students understand the important relationships between marketing, planning, operations, leadership, teamwork, and conflict management, all of which are essential to effective market and organization management.

The fourth case, "Intermountain Healthcare," is descriptive rather than decision oriented. It must be analyzed to understand the dynamics of the situation but does not require students to recommend action. This case profiles various elements of a model healthcare organization and invites students to consider a variety of questions and topics addressed in the text. Information for this case was derived from Intermountain Health-care's website (www.intermountainhealthcare.org).

The outline of the textbook, the cases, and our proposal of the five Ps for healthcare marketing efforts (patients, physicians, public, payers, and the presence of politics) come from our experiences working in the healthcare field, from teaching healthcare market-ing in the classroom, and from information gleaned from interviews conducted between 2009 and 2012 with a convenience sample ($n = 23$) of healthcare professionals engaged in marketing efforts. The respondents represent various healthcare marketing sites: clinics, for-profit and not-for-profit hospitals, physician practices, a long-term care facility, and an independent marketing/management contractor. They worked in a variety of loca-tions—the Southwest, the Southeast, the Northwest, the Intermountain West, and the Midwest—in both urban and rural settings. They also represent different positions of authority, from administrators in training in a physician clinic to regional directors of large hospitals (employing more than 50,000 people). Evident throughout this book are three themes that emerged from the interviews:

1. A commitment to and enthusiasm about their careers and the certainty that their work matters to the organization as well as to the larger community

2. A shared opinion that healthcare marketing is not general marketing in a different industry that just happens to be healthcare

3. A recommendation for instructors to underscore the importance of the patient, the physician, the payers, the public, and the presence of politics to students interested in healthcare marketing as a career

We hope that this book fills the need for a solid, undergraduate healthcare mar-keting text. And we hope that it "just fits" the need of our academic teaching colleagues who participated in the discussions held during the AUPHA workshop in 2008 and oth-ers who echo the sentiment. To that end, we have created instructor resources for this book. Ancillaries for each chapter include test questions and answers, PowerPoint slides, and sample answers to the end-of-chapter questions and end-of-chapter exercises. Also provided are teaching notes for the cases. For access to these resources, send an e-mail to hapbooks@ache.org.

Leigh W. Cellucci
Greenville, North Carolina

Carla Wiggins
Ogden, Utah

Tracy J. Farnsworth
Pocatello, Idaho

ACKNOWLEDGMENTS

We gratefully acknowledge the 23 healthcare professionals who gave up their time to tell us about their work. They exhibited commitment to and enthusiasm for their work and a love of the healthcare industry and the people they serve. From these interviews, we were able to identify the proposed five Ps for healthcare marketing efforts: physicians, payers, patients, public, and presence of politics. These professionals have asked to remain anonymous. We have honored their wishes, but we are indebted to them for their graciousness and willingness to share their work. Many of the case studies and end-of-chapter exercises were derived from the interviews. While the cases are disguised, all descriptions of events are factual.

Many of the case studies and end-of-chapter exercises were vetted in class or in round-table discussions at AUPHA conferences and workshops. In these meetings, we benefited from the comments of numerous individuals, particularly Dawn Oetjen, Reid Oetjen, Peter Fitzpatrick, and Mary Ann Keogh Hoss. In class, the health services management students at East Carolina University assessed (through in-class participation and feedback) which case studies and end-of-chapter exercises were worthy of print.

We also recognize and thank Tom Vitelli of Intermountain Healthcare and Paula Ginsborg of the California HealthCare Foundation. Their assistance in providing, reviewing, and approving material for use in the feature cases is deeply appreciated.

We appreciate as well the permission to reprint portions of writing that were originally published elsewhere, including the American Health Information Management Association

(AHIMA) Standards of Ethical Coding. We also acknowledge the Academy of Management for permission conveyed through Copyright Clearance Center to reprint the table regarding dimension of organizational politics from Mayes, B. and W. Allen. 1977. "Toward a Definition of Organizational Politics." *Academy of Management Review* 2 (4): 675.

Throughout our work on this text, we have benefited greatly from the collegial support of Michael Kennedy, Susie Harris, Elizabeth Forrestal, Bob Kulesher, Thomas Ross, Myra Brown, Robert Campbell, Paul Bell, Patricia Royal, Bonita Sasnett, Jennifer Pitt, and Rosa Harris. Additionally, Xiaoming Zeng, chair of the Department of Health Services and Information Management in the College of Allied Health Sciences at East Carolina University, deserves special mention for his continued support.

Finally, we acknowledge the professionals at Health Administration Press. Eileen Lynch, Carrie McDonald, and Janet Davis served as our acquisitions editors. Their support of our work on an undergraduate text for healthcare marketing was unwavering. We especially thank them for their patience and guidance. They worked with three different authors at three different sites in different time zones, yet they did so with solid professionalism and good humor. Jennifer Seibert served as our senior editor, and we appreciate her expert attention to detail and careful read of our drafts.

On a personal note, Leigh W. Cellucci thanks her family: her husband, Tony, for his constant support, solid advice, and love; her sons, Vincent and Robert; her daughter, Kimberly; and her son-in-law, Daniel. Their support and encouragement are indeed treasured.

Carla Wiggins thanks her adopted brothers and sisters—Mary, Jim, Pat, Linda, and Mary Kay—for their love and caring. And, as always, she thanks Mark for his support and encouragement and for enriching her life beyond what words can express.

Tracy Farnsworth gratefully acknowledges his dear wife, Michelle; Linda Hatzenbuehler, executive dean of the Division of Health Sciences at Idaho State University; and coauthors Leigh W. Cellucci and Carla Wiggins. After 23 eventful years in healthcare management, Michelle's, Linda's, Leigh's, and Carla's invitations, mentoring, and support enabled his joyful and productive transition to higher education.

PART I

FOUNDATIONS OF HEALTHCARE MARKETING

This real-life case invites students to consider the dynamic relationship healthcare providers have with their local and regional market and to appreciate the need to balance organizational and community interests when making important decisions that affect the healthcare marketplace. Participant and facility names and various numerical values have been modified to preserve anonymity and accentuate points of learning.

The case also encourages students to consider the long-term impact certain strategic initiatives have on healthcare organizations and their stakeholders, including patients, physicians, payers, and the public, and to actively consider stakeholder expectations in connection with these decisions. Finally, this case introduces students to important healthcare industry issues and trends, including forces that shape a healthcare organization's mission, vision, and market-based strategies for growth and development, as discussed in Part I of this text.

INTRODUCTION

In many ways the 2001 holiday season was no different than any other. Dallin Call—chief executive officer of Kimball Hospital—genuinely enjoyed the traditional music, decorations, and seemingly endless social gatherings characteristic of the time of year. It was dissimilar in one respect, however: Dallin was full of anxiety and could not shake it. Three months earlier, Dallin's Rocky Mountain–based healthcare system—Great Western Hospital Corporation (GWHC)—initiated merger/consolidation talks with the county-based operators of his hospital's chief rival, Tanner Medical Center, and a December 31 deadline to formally initiate negotiations or walk away was looming. Dallin understood that his personal recommendation to his corporate supervisors and community-based board would greatly influence their eventual decision to press ahead with consolidation talks or continue the more than 40-year practice of offering competitive but duplicative healthcare services to the community. Dallin's recommendation and the ultimate decision to consolidate or not would be the most important local healthcare market decision in a generation or more and would greatly impact the lives of numerous healthcare professionals and the nature and quality of healthcare services for area residents for years to come.

MERGER AND CONSOLIDATION TRENDS

In general, the local market mirrored the healthcare issues and challenges observed nationally, including a trend toward hospital mergers, acquisitions, and consolidations brought about by myriad organizational and market forces (Cuellar and Gertler 2003; Haleblian et al. 2009). In the decade preceding GWHC's deliberations, the healthcare industry underwent a wave of consolidations that transformed the hospital marketplace. By the mid-1990s, hospital mergers and acquisitions had increased by nearly tenfold the rate observed only five years earlier (Vogt and Town 2006).

From his readings and observations, Dallin noted that some of the more important advantages to hospital mergers and consolidations included much needed access to capital and elimination of non-value-added duplication of expensive healthcare services. Mindful that consolidation was rarely a panacea, however, Dallin identified a handful of concerns and potential disadvantages, including the potential for higher costs and prices and lower quality following reduced competition (Tenn 2011; Vogt and Town 2006).

THE LOCAL MARKET AND DEMOGRAPHICS

Prattville's high desert community of 50,000 generally supported two competing hospitals for more than 70 years. About 75 percent of one hospital's clinical programs and services were duplicated by its cross-town rival, and local citizens traveled to out-of-area hospitals to receive roughly $40 million per year in healthcare services either not provided or poorly delivered by local hospitals.

From early 2000 through mid-2001, important changes in the leadership and governance of Prattville's rival hospitals set the stage for the important talks that soon followed. Among these leadership changes was the appointment of new hospital board chairmen, new hospital administrators/CEOs, new Blade County commissioners, and new regional and systemwide leadership at GWHC. Moreover, each hospital's respective plans to introduce an even greater array of duplicate services or expand on existing duplicate services prompted Dallin to ask himself three important questions: Was his hospital's mission focused on what was right and best for the Prattville community or GWHC? Would a consolidation of hospital operations improve Prattville area residents' access to services and the cost and quality of healthcare? And which organization—Kimball Hospital (GWHC) or county-owned/operated Tanner Medical Center—was best positioned to assume leadership, ownership, and management of the community's hospital/healthcare system?

Mindful of the sea change in local and central office leadership and increasingly troubled by an awareness that each hospital's strategic plan called for more and more non-value-added duplication of hospital services, Dallin contacted his immediate supervisor and suggested the time might be right to revisit the idea of hospital cooperation—even consolidation. The most recent serious attempt at merger/consolidation talks failed in 1983, and authorities revisited the idea in 1990 without success. When merger/consolidation talks resurfaced in 2001, GWHC was ever mindful of its longstanding, publicly stated commitment to the community. Yet GWHC was cognizant of important political and marketplace realities. A profile of key ownership, market, financial, operating, and political dimensions of Prattville's hospital/healthcare community is presented in Exhibit 1.

OTHER PROVIDER AND COMMUNITY CONSIDERATIONS

Since its inception in 1975, GWHC had established a system of more than 20 hospitals in three neighboring states with highly sophisticated central office support services, including health information technology, central purchasing, laboratory, laundry, marketing/advertising, physician recruitment, quality/risk management, and more. By implementing evidence-based medicine, the system had reduced costs and improved quality and received national acclaim for its remarkable focus on this initiative.

Because of its local ownership and control, employees and supporters of Tanner Medical Center touted the hospital's ability to chart its own course and make its own decisions, independent of out-of-state officers who may or may not have shared the community's healthcare goals and views. Tanner Medical Center enjoyed a measure of "system" support through its affiliation with Voluntary Hospitals of America (VHA), the nation's largest not-for-profit hospital association. Importantly, and for a combination of reasons, local physicians generally favored and supported Tanner over Kimball, reflected by a nearly 2:1 ratio of annual patient admissions to Tanner over Kimball. Many supposed that notwithstanding Kimball's/GWHC's reputation as a high-quality, lower-cost provider, area physicians resisted the corporation's centralized, systematic approach to planning and

	Kimball Hospital	Tanner Medical Center
Hospital ownership and control	GWHC	Blade County
Ownership type	501(c)(3) corporation	Government/county
Licensed beds	110	150
Total patient days—trend (1998/1999/2000)	10,150/10,925/12,775	24,240/25,380/23,725
Average daily census	35	68
Annual gross patient services revenue	$49 million	$97 million
Annual net patient services revenue	$31.5 million	$54.6 million
Market share	26%	52%
Annual marketing/ advertising budget	$141,000	$310,000
Net operating income percentage—trend (1998/1999/2000)	3%/5%/3%	2%/4%/6%
Total debt	N/A (consolidated with GWHC)	$73 million
Financial reserves (savings)	$2.3 billion (GWHC)	$9 million
Employed physicians	8	0
Percentage of local physicians whose first loyalty was to this hospital	35%	65%
Services unique to hospital in local market	Cardiology, acute rehabilitation	Pediatrics, neonatal level II, cancer
Percentage of physicians who favored hospital consolidation	80% (based on fall 2001 survey of Kimball/Tanner medical staffs)	
Public preference for local (versus out of area) ownership and control	68% (based on spring 2001 Kimball Hospital community telephone survey)	

delivering patient care. Indeed, many physicians relocated to Prattville because of the region's laissez-faire approach to medicine, including a lack of managed care and other insurance mechanisms that limited physician reimbursement and autonomy.

A TIME FOR DECISION

As CEO, Dallin was also chief marketing manager and promoter of his hospital/healthcare organization. Positioning his organization for immediate and long-term growth and financial success was an ever-present mandate; orchestrating a well-balanced, integrated, community-wide healthcare system to improve access, cost, and quality of care to the entire Prattville community was no less important. In his heart, Dallin believed the time was right to consolidate or merge the community's two competing hospitals, and the leadership, financial, and other strengths of his company made Kimball Hospital/GWHC the preferred owner/operator of the new entity. Yet, Dallin knew of his community's underlying preference for local ownership and control and of the physician community's long-standing reluctance to embrace his company's philosophy and approach to organizing and delivering care. Although Dallin's organization and community board leaders were independent, critical thinkers, they looked to him for guidance in this matter.

DISCUSSION QUESTIONS

1. What key organizational and marketplace issues reopened the door to a potential hospital merger/consolidation?
2. In what ways could Dallin balance the interests of the community with the interests of his employer/corporation?
3. From a patient and community perspective, what might be some of the pros and cons to consolidating the community's hospitals?
4. From this case, can you identify and describe some of the forces that shape a hospital's mission, vision, culture, growth, and development?
5. Who are the key decision makers and other stakeholders (individuals and groups) in this case? What issues and concerns do they have about consolidation, and what are their relative positions of power and influence in Prattville's healthcare community?
6. Would you recommend consolidation of Prattville's two community hospitals? Why or why not?
7. If you would recommend consolidation, which organization should assume ownership/control? Why? What would be the strategic marketing implications of your decision?

REFERENCES

Cuellar, A. E., and P. J. Gertler. 2003. "Trends in Hospital Consolidation: The Formation of Local Systems." *Health Affairs (Millwood)* 22 (6): 77–87.

Haleblian, J., C. E. Devers, G. McNamara, M. A. Carpenter, and R. B. Davison. 2009. "Taking Stock of What We Know About Mergers and Acquisitions." *Journal of Management* 35 (3): 469–502.

Tenn, S. 2011. "The Price Effects of Hospital Mergers: A Case Study of the Sutter-Summit Transaction." *International Journal of the Economics of Business* 18 (1) 65–82.

Vogt, W. B., and R. Town. 2006. "How Has Hospital Consolidation Affected the Price and Quality of Hospital Care?" Robert Wood Johnson Foundation Research Synthesis Report No. 9. Published in February. www.rwjf.org/content/dam/farm/reports/issue_briefs/2006/rwjf12056/subassets/rwjf12056_1.

CHAPTER 1

THE HEALTHCARE INDUSTRY AND HEALTHCARE MARKETING

After studying this chapter, you will be able to

➤ describe the history, size, and diversity of the US healthcare industry;

➤ demonstrate a rudimentary understanding of health insurance and reimbursement mechanisms; and

➤ explain how the fundamentals of market competition do/do not work in US healthcare.

CASE STUDY: WHAT IS HEALTHCARE ADMINISTRATION ANYWAY?

Sarah Creek was excited. After a year of studies at the local university, she had finally found her major: healthcare administration (HCA). It was just what she had been looking for! She knew she wanted to spend her life in a discipline that served others, but she really did not want to be part of direct patient care. She first had thought she might major in business, and for a while that idea felt right. But the more she thought about it, the more she felt that she didn't want to dedicate herself to working for companies whose only goal was selling more "things" and making more profit; she wanted something more. When a new friend at a party mentioned he was an HCA major, Sarah was intrigued.

When she told her parents and friends about her exciting decision, they reacted skeptically. Were there any jobs for HCA majors? Didn't HCA majors need a nursing or medical background? What exactly did a healthcare manager do? Where would she work? Was she going to spend her life working in a hospital? What about all of those unflattering, confrontational, money-centered administrators featured in hospital dramas on television—was that the type of person she wanted to become?

Sarah was not thinking along those lines at all, and their perceptions did not sound anything like her friend's description of HCA, so Sarah made an appointment with an HCA professor to talk about the major and the field. While chatting with the professor, she learned about the size and diversity of healthcare settings and facilities. They talked about the many disciplines within the field of healthcare administration, such as finance, human resources management, and marketing. They also talked about related industries, such as pharmaceuticals, durable medical equipment, medical transportation, health insurance, and health education and promotion. The combinations and opportunities seemed nearly endless. By the time she left the professor's office, Sarah was certain she would be able to find her place in the huge, wide-ranging field of HCA and was ready and eager to answer her family's and friends' questions.

HEALTHCARE DELIVERY IN THE UNITED STATES

third-party payer
the third entity involved in health services transactions, after the provider (first) and the patient (second) (A health insurance company is one example of a third-party payer.)

From birth to death, nearly everyone in the United States has some contact and interaction with the healthcare industry. Consisting of hospitals, clinics, and nursing homes; pharmaceuticals, medical equipment, and information technology; physicians, nurses, therapists, technicians, and managers; and all the facilities, **third-party payers**, businesses, and personnel in between, the US healthcare industry is arguably the largest, most complex, and most pervasive industry in the nation and, perhaps, the world.

What started in the 1700s as a small cottage industry of mostly apprentice-trained solo practitioners, volunteer nurses, and almshouses for the poor has grown into today's huge, fragmented, and highly sophisticated health and medical care enterprise. One could say that the United States has not just one healthcare industry but an array of interconnected health and medical industries, each with its own technology, target populations, treatments, consumers, and personnel.

Consider, for example, what many people think of as the traditional healthcare industry: hospitals. Most people don't know about the high level of competition among facilities, the tight profit margins reported by some and the large profits reported by others, the high level of liability involved, the complexity of reimbursement for patient care, and the high cost of personnel and administration in this particular part of US healthcare. Even this best-known—and somewhat taken for granted—segment of healthcare can be parsed into public and private sectors, urban and rural locations, large and small facilities, specialty care and primary care, and specific types of patients and diseases. Many simply assume that all hospitals provide the entire range of treatment options to everyone and that hospitals have to admit and care for all patients who enter their doors, regardless of ability to pay. Those inside the industry know that nearly every one of these assumptions is false.

Another example is the **ambulatory care** side of healthcare. It consists of physician offices and clinics; freestanding and hospital-affiliated emergency and urgent care providers; surgery centers, pharmacies, dental offices, and therapy/rehabilitation clinics; and psychologists, counselors, and other mental and behavioral health practitioners, to name just a few. Ambulatory care and other healthcare sectors significantly overlap. A case in point is pharmacies; they are certainly part of ambulatory care but also are part of the huge, expensive pharmaceutical industry, which carries out basic bench research on treatments and medicines, conducts clinical trials, and engages in ubiquitous drug advertising. Without the high-tech pharmaceutical industry and its thousands of over-the-counter and prescription medications, many people would live shorter, more painful, and more disease-ridden lives.

Yet another part of the healthcare industry focuses on the elderly and their needs. Senior housing, senior-living communities, assisted living, and **long-term care** facilities most often come to mind, but home health care is a large part of this industry segment, as are pharmaceuticals, durable medical equipment, adult day care, hospice, rehabilitation, respite care, and nutrition. Diet and nutrition are in themselves large, dynamic industries. They include large, for-profit weight loss programs, facility kitchens and cafeterias, vitamins, food supplements, organic foods, exercise, health clubs, and spas.

The sectors mentioned thus far are barely a scratch on the surface. There are sides of healthcare few people ever think about: information technology, health education and literacy, medical transportation, medical equipment and technology manufacturing, and public health, among others.

One such side of healthcare is the system of education for health professionals: physicians, nurses, therapists, technicians, information specialists, and managers. Medical schools, schools of public health, colleges of health professions, nursing schools, community colleges, and universities play a vital role in our national and personal health. They compete against

ambulatory care
healthcare services that do not require an overnight stay in a hospital; also called *outpatient care*

long-term care
an array of services, both medical and nonmedical, for people who need help over long periods; often associated with nursing homes

each other for students and for funding and research grants but are often an overlooked, yet absolutely crucial, part of healthcare. And there is the sometimes famous, sometimes infamous health insurance industry, from private insurance firms to the huge government programs of Medicare and Medicaid, the Indian Health Service, Maternal and Child Health, the Veterans Administration, and the myriad state and local programs across the United States.

Clearly, discussion of the many industries that fall under the umbrella of healthcare could go on and on. There is a point to this litany: Each has its own needs and message to share, and each needs to be profitable enough to survive.

TRENDS IN HEALTHCARE DELIVERY

sliding fee scale
a reimbursement system that uses an individual's income, financial resources, and ability to pay as the basis for determining the amount he or she will pay for a healthcare service

Long before anyone thought of healthcare as an industry, solo practitioners tended to the illnesses and health needs of the people in their communities. **Sliding fee scales**, reimbursement systems, and malpractice insurance did not exist. Doctors came to the patient's home, provided what care and comfort they could, and were often paid whatever the patient or family could afford. Hospitals as we think of them today also did not exist. The hospitals that did exist were not places to go to be cured and made whole; they were places only the poorest of the poor went to die. Anyone who had family or money was taken care of in the home. As the United States entered the 1900s, hospitals began to change, primarily due to the great advances in science that were occurring worldwide. From the late-1800s to the mid-1900s, the introduction of germ theory, the discovery of vitamins and insulin, the introduction of food safety standards and waste management, and the widespread accomplishments of vaccination programs led the way to understanding the disease process and, in turn, to the development of effective prevention measures and treatments for many diseases and illnesses. This new belief in science provided a firm foundation for what we now think of as the healthcare industry.

Until the time of the Great Depression, the US government saw no role for itself in the personal health and well-being of US citizens. The Great Depression's unprecedented unemployment, homelessness, and suffering provided the impetus for one of the United States' first government programs: Social Security. At first, Social Security provided no benefits specific to healthcare, but it did set a precedent for the government's later involvement in caring and providing for the health of US citizens.

In times of economic downturn, the demand and need for health services and medical care do not necessarily decrease; one might argue that bad economic times actually create the need for more health services and medical care. Hospitals, which had evolved into true treatment centers by the time of the Great Depression, faced a dilemma: Their missions called for them to care for the people in their communities, yet many people seeking their services had no means to pay for care. How could hospitals continue to provide care to their patients for free and still manage to bring in enough revenue to pay their own bills and remain open? The cliché "no margin, no mission" became an everyday challenge for hospitals across the country.

Baylor Hospital in Texas is most often credited with finding a solution to this dilemma by establishing a new way for patients to pay for their medical care. The hospital asked each faculty member at Baylor University to pay a small, predetermined amount per month, and in return the hospital provided all the care that faculty member needed in that month. This prepaid approach to care was a win–win solution for everyone. It reduced individuals' financial uncertainty because they would incur no bills if they needed to be hospitalized. People could budget an exact amount for medical care each month, and they knew that regardless of the hospital care they might need, it would be provided at no additional cost. Furthermore, it reduced Baylor Hospital's financial **risk** because it had a certain, regular, prepaid flow of income each month. Not every person who prepaid would need care every month, and the hospital would be able to use some of that prepaid income to cover the costs of care for those who could not pay. This innovation was the birth of health insurance and what we now know as the US healthcare industry.

Prepaid healthcare, aka health insurance, really came into its own after World War II. The US government was surprised by the number of young men who had not been able to be enlisted in the armed services due to physical/health deficiencies. These men were predominantly in their late teens to late twenties, a time when they should have been in their prime. The government's concern over this issue was threefold. First, the inability of so many men to serve in the military was a realistic security concern. Second was the concern that many men with health and physical problems would not be able to fully participate in, and contribute to, the nation's workforce, productivity, and long-term economic advancement. Finally, for moral and ethical reasons, perhaps the government did have a responsibility to help ensure US citizens' health and well-being. To address these concerns, the federal government created three federal programs. It established the National Institutes of Health to research and find cures for diseases; passed the Hill-Burton Act, which offered low-interest loans to communities to build hospitals and clinics; and assigned health insurance tax-exempt status, which provided that neither employers nor employees would pay tax on the money employers used to purchase health insurance for their employees.

Through the creation and implementation of all three programs, the federal government's role in them was indirect; it created an environment in which US citizens could live healthier and more productive lives but did not actually provide care directly. Assignment of tax-exempt status to health insurance in particular did just what the federal government wanted it to do: It created a strong incentive for employers to provide health insurance for their employees and for employees to have their health insurance purchased for them with pretax money from their employers. Thus, in the post–World War II United States, employer-purchased health insurance became the predominant payment mechanism for health services and medical care.

The large-scale health insurance industry that developed in the United States reimbursed hospitals and physicians on a fee-for-service, **retrospective** basis, which is referred to as the *usual, customary, and reasonable (UCR)* reimbursement system. The amount the provider receives is decided *after* the service has been delivered. After providing care to the

risk
uncertainty

retrospective reimbursement
payment system in which the amount the provider is reimbursed is decided by the insurance company after the service has been rendered

patient, the hospital or physician submits an itemized bill requesting reimbursement from the patient's health insurance carrier. Upon receiving the request for reimbursement, the insurance company determines whether the requested amount is within the usual range of charges for those services and within the range of reimbursement the insurance company customarily remits for those services and then decides whether it is reasonable to pay the provider the amount requested. Reimbursement requests are *unbundled*—listed piece by piece and service by service—because it is more profitable for the provider to request reimbursement for each and every small segment of care and service delivered than to count all care rendered as one service (i.e., bundle) and request reimbursement for just that one bundle. Finally, because UCR reimbursement does not have a preset fee schedule, providers could steadily increase the amount of reimbursement they requested and thus raise the UCR reimbursement intervals higher and higher.

By the time Medicare and Medicaid were created in the mid-1960s, the UCR reimbursement system was firmly engrained and became the payment mechanism for these two public programs. By the 1970s, however, Medicare and Medicaid had grown into hugely expensive programs, and government at both the state and federal level began to question the wisdom of UCR reimbursement, which had allowed healthcare costs to rise much faster than the pace of inflation. The healthcare industry seemed to be spinning out of control. Health technology had become a double-edged sword: While paving the way for hospitals to become science fiction–like miracle factories, new technologies were rapidly being developed and used and often were implemented before their true costs and benefits were thoroughly analyzed. The number of health professions had exploded, each with its own education system and licensing requirements. Many thought that healthcare had simply become too big and too expensive to sustain.

In the 1972 presidential election, each candidate clearly needed to have a healthcare plank in his platform. The Democrats continued to champion national health insurance. The Republicans needed a healthcare initiative distinct from national health insurance, and thus they introduced health maintenance organizations (HMOs). The Republican candidate, Richard Nixon, won the election, and soon thereafter Congress passed the HMO Act, which provided start-up monies for these new organizations.

HMOs and managed care are beautiful in theory. On paper they effectively reverse all the perverse financial incentives of the UCR system and promote a true health-oriented approach to care. In practice, however, managed care became rigid, restricting hospital care and reimbursing only for preapproved services from specific HMO providers. Still, many HMO patients had more favorable health outcomes at a lower cost than did patients with traditional fee-for-service health insurance, and HMOs and managed care evolved and grew in the private health insurance sector.

Throughout the 1970s, a number of cost control mechanisms were introduced in an attempt to control Medicare costs and spending. None of them was successful at staunching the apparently unlimited need and demand for healthcare services among the nation's elderly. Thus, in 1983 Medicare introduced a new payment system for hospitals called *Diagnosis-Related Groups (DRGs)*, a prospective, fee schedule approach that reimbursed predetermined amounts by diagnosis, not by each service provided. In a **prospective payment** system, providers know *before* the service is rendered the amount the insurance company will reimburse. While this approach may sound reasonable today, in 1983 it was earth-shattering. For many services, hospitals did not know how much they spent on patients; they counted on being generously reimbursed by insurance and then cost shifting some of the over-reimbursement to cover services they provided free of charge to those unable to pay. Cost shifting was a virtually unknown practice unless one was a hospital CEO or CFO. It did, however, enable hospitals to meet their broad missions of caring for the poor and the uninsured.

prospective payment
reimbursement system in which providers know *before* the service is rendered the amount the insurance company will cover

The introduction of DRGs and other prospective reimbursement mechanisms forced providers to become far more financially sophisticated and fiscally responsible. Medicare reimbursement was a large segment of most hospitals' and physicians' revenue. Providers soon found that when reimbursement was strictly limited to a predetermined amount, they could remain viable only if they eliminated waste and allocated all resources wisely to every service provided to each and every customer. Inevitably certain services became recognized as far more profitable than others and certain customers became far less profitable than others. For the first time in its history, the healthcare industry needed to think about what it was providing, how it was providing it, and to whom it was providing it. In this way, the healthcare industry slowly and painfully adopted a competitive, market-oriented approach to seeking and caring for customers.

The Challenges of a Competitive Market

The US economy is predominantly a **market-based economy**. Nearly all US market transactions and exchanges are based on the rudiments of supply and demand. The more closely an industry adheres to the following five fundamentals of the competitive market, the more competitive the market and the better supply and demand performs in that industry:

market-based economy
a system of production and consumption of goods and services in which transactions and exchanges are based on the rudiments of supply and demand and fundamental competitive principles

1. Buyers have complete product knowledge.

2. Buyers are free to purchase from any seller.

3. Sellers are free to enter and exit the market.

4. No collusion or price setting exists among sellers.

5. Prices are set solely by supply and demand.

One can reasonably argue that none of these five market tenets truly exists in its purest form in today's global markets. However, the US healthcare industry is particularly egregious in this respect. The implication here is not that the economic laws of the market don't work in healthcare; they do. The competitive market in healthcare is just not as intuitively obvious as it is in other industries.

For example, how do hospitals compete for physicians? How do physicians and hospitals compete for customers? While physicians might be able to induce demand for services such as checkups and elective surgery, can physicians compete or create demand for coronary bypass surgery? How can hospitals ensure that they have only the best physicians on staff? How can patients have complete product knowledge in an industry so advanced that even providers in one specialty don't understand the product or service offered by those in another? How can a seriously ill or injured person reasonably shop for and decide which physician will provide the best care at the most affordable cost? When an insurance company or HMO restricts reimbursement to its panel of providers and that insurance is purchased by an employer, how can employees covered by that insurance be free to purchase services from any seller or provider?

Perhaps an even more perplexing question in regard to healthcare is, who are the true buyers and sellers of health services? Is the customer the insurance company that is reimbursing/paying for the services? Is the customer the employer who is choosing and purchasing the insurance? Is the customer the insured patient who is likely paying for some portion of the cost of the care provided? Likewise, similar questions can be asked about the seller. Is the physician the seller? Is the physician's group practice or the hospital the seller? Is the insurance company that works to steer its members to certain providers and certain types of services the seller? So, returning to the original question posed earlier, how should healthcare providers and healthcare facilities compete?

HEALTHCARE MARKETING DEFINED

The complexity of the competitive market in healthcare compels healthcare managers and leaders to study and master the art of healthcare marketing. Healthcare marketing is not just placing advertisements and searching for more customers. Healthcare marketing is not creating demand for extra, sometimes unnecessary, expensive services so facilities can make more money. Healthcare marketing is a fine-tuned art and science that creates, communicates, and delivers offerings that have value for healthcare stakeholders.

This text discusses how healthcare administrators, public relations officers, clinic managers, and marketing directors (or whatever job title they hold) create, communicate, and deliver services that have value for healthcare patients, physicians, the public, and payers. Their focus is on these five Ps: patients, physicians, the public, payers, and the presence of politics. For example, the book discusses how a for-profit hospital used marketing to inform the public (and potential patients) about its new surgical technology—the daVinci robot. For those in the community who require surgery for coronary artery disease, it is valuable to know that this service—minimally invasive surgery for a complex surgical procedure—is available at their local hospital. The book also shows how a community health center administrator targeted marketing efforts to a specific group—Medicaid-eligible individuals—to let them know that the center's providers spoke both English and Spanish. For those who have Medicaid and do not speak English well, knowledge that they can actually converse with their doctor in their native language is not only valuable—it also can be lifesaving.

CHAPTER QUESTIONS

1. What forces changed US healthcare from a cottage-based, loose network of apprentice-trained providers into the large, high-tech industry it is today?
2. Provide examples of retrospective and prospective reimbursement, and distinguish between them.
3. What is healthcare marketing, and what is its role in today's healthcare industry?

CHAPTER EXERCISES

1. *We need to advertise, don't we?*

   It is said that in the United States, one-third of all heart bypass surgeries are clearly unneeded, one-third are questionable, and one-third are clearly needed. Another widely accepted adage is that the vast majority of patients in the United States receive either too much care or too little care; few receive the exact amount of care they truly need. How does healthcare marketing contribute to these problems? Propose a way for healthcare marketing to address these issues.

2. *Who really purchases healthcare?*

   This chapter introduces important questions regarding the true buyers, sellers, and customers in the US healthcare industry. Who do you believe to be the true purchaser of healthcare in the United States? Prepare a four-paragraph persuasive argument supporting your answer, formatted as directed in the following list. Choose only one purchaser, not a number or combination of purchasers.

   ➤ Paragraph 1: State who you believe to be the true purchaser of healthcare in the United States, and provide two solid reasons for your answer.

   ➤ Paragraph 2: Expand on your first reason for believing that the entity you named in paragraph 1 is the true purchaser.

➤ Paragraph 3: Expand on your second reason for believing that the entity you named in paragraph 1 is the true purchaser.

➤ Paragraph 4: Reiterate your belief, and conclude your argument.

CHAPTER 2

THE GROWTH OF MARKETING EFFORTS IN HEALTHCARE

After studying this chapter, you will be able to

➤ explain the history of marketing in healthcare,

➤ discuss how the marketing/public relations department fits into the larger healthcare organization, and

➤ describe the healthcare "customer."

CASE STUDY: THE AMERICAN MARKETING ASSOCIATION, HAWORTH PRESS, AND MARKETING EFFORTS IN HEALTHCARE

Marketing in the healthcare arena has grown primarily because of three factors: changing healthcare policy, changing consumer expectations, and changing attitudes regarding the stigma of marketing by the healthcare profession. Accompanying these changes was the evolution of journals that focused on healthcare marketing. This case describes the history of academic and professional publications as they pertain to healthcare marketing and illustrates how the study of healthcare marketing evolved.

Academic studies, reports from marketing events in healthcare organizations, and theories about marketing as it applied to healthcare were published to help professionals learn about and practice marketing in healthcare. It took time for marketing to earn its place as an accepted part of the healthcare arena. Simply put, prior to the 1970s most hospitals did not have a marketing department, nor did they employ a person titled "director of marketing," "director of public relations," "vice president of public relations," or "chief marketing officer."

Marketing had not earned its place at the table in strategic planning, decision making, and budget allocation when the American Marketing Association published the first issue of the *Journal of Health Care Marketing* (*JHCM*) in 1980. In *JHCM*'s first "From the Editors" column, B. J. Dunlap and Don Dodson (1980–1981, 4), founding editors of the journal, wrote that the purpose of the journal was to "serve as a bridge between the academicians and the practitioners who have an interest in marketing for nonprofit organizations, specifically focusing on that which is of a health care nature."

In 1983, Haworth Press, publisher of scholarly articles on healthcare and social, information, and library sciences, issued *Health Marketing Quarterly*, a journal focused on the marketing of group practices. Its founding editor, William J. Winston, emphasized that its articles were practical and written for practitioners. Four years later, Haworth published the *Journal of Hospital Marketing*, which was designed as an applied journal—that is, a journal "for practitioners, and by practitioners" (Winston 1986, 1). Both of Haworth's journals were founded by Winston, who had an unwavering commitment to marketing's legitimate place in healthcare.

Changes were made to all three journals throughout their publication history. *JHCM*'s name was changed to *Marketing Health Services* in 1997, and the *Journal of Hospital Marketing* became the *Journal of Hospital Marketing and Public Relations* in 2002. In 2007, Haworth Press was bought out by the Taylor and Francis Group, and the *Journal of Hospital Marketing and Public Relations* was placed under the auspices of Routledge. Finally, in 2010, *Health Marketing Quarterly* incorporated the *Journal of Hospital Marketing and Public Relations*. Today, the American Marketing Association publishes *Marketing Health Services* and Routledge publishes *Health Marketing Quarterly*. Both journals remain focused on marketing issues in healthcare, featuring articles, commentaries, case studies, and tools for healthcare marketing professionals.

Along with the success of these journals, the practice of marketing in healthcare also earned acceptance as part of the healthcare arena. Simply put, hospitals became accustomed to employing a director of marketing, director of public relations, vice president of public relations, or chief marketing officer, and marketing earned its place at the table in strategic planning, decision making, and budget allocation.

Changes in healthcare policy, healthcare consumers' expectations, and attitudes about marketing by the healthcare profession all helped to bring about this acceptance. Today it is common practice for people to receive a text reminding them that their prescription is ready; make an appointment through physician practices', clinics', and hospitals' websites; receive pamphlets about proper nutrition for persons with diabetes; and be surveyed about their outpatient surgery experience. All of these marketing efforts have been discussed, criticized, and refined via various avenues, including the journals featured in this case study.

THE HISTORY OF MARKETING IN HEALTHCARE
DEFINING HEALTHCARE MARKETING

The focus of **healthcare marketing** is meeting the needs of patients, physicians, the public, and payers. The American Marketing Association (2007) defines *marketing* as "the activity, set of institutions, and processes for creating, communicating, delivering, and exchanging offerings that have value for customers, clients, partners, and society at large." The definition of *healthcare marketing* was built on this definition. As stated in Chapter 1, healthcare marketing is a fine-tuned art and science that creates, communicates, and delivers offerings that have **value** for healthcare stakeholders. It is important to note that healthcare marketing does not exist in a vacuum. Professionals who work in healthcare marketing departments are part of the strategic team, whether a large team assembled for hospital-based initiatives or a small team formed for clinic-based projects.

For example, a physician clinic may employ the best-trained, smartest physicians, but if the environment is off-putting, patients may choose to go elsewhere for care. Even though meeting patients' clinical needs is the most important outcome of a physician–patient encounter, research indicates that the environment of a physician's office also has an impact on the patients' total care experience (Altringer 2010; Bitner 1992; Fottler et al. 2000). Dr. Mary Jo Bitner, a professor and researcher recognized as one of the founders and pioneers in the field of service marketing and management, presented the health clinic as a service organization that performs actions within an environment of elaborate physical complexity. As such, the service scape of the clinic should focus on eliciting a desired response from patients. Bitner (1992, 64) asked

healthcare marketing
a fine-tuned art and science that creates, communicates, and delivers offerings that have value for healthcare stakeholders, including patients, physicians, the public, and payers

value
relative worth; quality received in exchange for an investment of time, money, or effort

[I]n the case of the hospital, what beliefs, emotions, and physiological responses will encourage patients to get up and walk around the facility if that is the desired behavior for their recovery?

Architecture is one way to communicate value to patients. The floor plan, placement of furniture, and room decor all contribute to the image of the clinic (e.g., professional, clean) and the quality of its service (e.g., the ease of navigating the designed space, providers' diplomas on the walls).

healthscape
the service areas, waiting rooms, and architecture of a healthcare organization (e.g., physician's office, hospital atrium) that reinforce to patients the high quality of care they will experience

Dr. Myron Fottler, professor of health services administration and executive director of health services administration programs at the University of Central Florida, and colleagues (2000, 101) used the term **healthscape** to define service areas that meet or exceed patients' needs and reinforce the quality of care. For instance, Mayo Clinic has an atrium featuring a grand piano that anyone is welcome to play. The daughter of one Mayo patient described the atrium as a place where people come "to heal together and share what brings [them] hope and joy" (Hume 2009). The value delivered by the healthscape of Mayo Clinic is part of what marketing is all about.

However, healthcare administrators and providers in hospitals, clinics, and other settings did not always use or condone marketing in healthcare. In fact, marketing's history in healthcare can be traced back to discussions in the field of marketing during the late 1960s. Philip Kotler, known as the "father of social marketing," and Sidney J. Levy (1969), recognized as one of the main contributors to the field of marketing and consumer behavior in the twentieth century, proposed that the concept of marketing be broadened to arenas outside of the sale of products, such as toothpaste, soap, and steel (10). They emphasized that the marketing concept of serving and satisfying human needs fits well with the purpose of hospitals—serving the sick and satisfying the health needs of consumers. Dodson (1985) asserted that marketing was introduced into the healthcare field when Kotler (1975) extended this line of thought, proposing that the basics of general marketing (e.g., distributing information to educate, motivate, and service target markets) applied to healthcare. The case study at the beginning of this chapter mentioned that today, customers receive texts notifying them that their prescriptions are ready, indicating that pharmacies have clearly adopted Kotler's stance and engage in marketing activities such as texting to serve its market and satisfy its customers' health needs.

THE EVOLUTION OF MARKETING IN HEALTHCARE

As stated at the beginning of this chapter's case study, marketing in healthcare has grown primarily because of changes in healthcare policy, consumers' expectations, and attitudes about marketing by the healthcare profession. Let's examine these three factors.

Changes in Healthcare Policy

As discussed in Chapter 1, healthcare policy began to change in the 1970s. Payment shifted from primarily UCR reimbursement to include cost containment mechanisms, such as DRGs and HMOs. This shift brought hospitals and clinics to consider the importance of knowing what services they provided, how they provided them, and who received them. After the introduction of predetermined fee schedules for reimbursement, healthcare providers were reimbursed more for some services than they were for other services and, over time, turned to marketing as a tool to help them create communications to educate and promote their services to prospective patients. In 1986, Winston stated that changing payment mechanisms had the greatest impact on healthcare marketing (26). The term *easy money* was used in publications to refer to payment structures prior to the introduction of cost containment policies (Clarke 1978; Gavin 1980–1981). Roberta Clarke (1978), associate professor at Boston University's School of Management and former president of the Society for Healthcare Planning and Marketing, proposed that the availability of easy money in the 1960s allowed for unregulated, unmonitored growth of health centers, which did not consider that this easy money could disappear. Marshall P. Gavin, president of Primecare Corporation, a company that provided marketing services for medical centers, asserted in a guest editorial for the *Journal of Health Care Marketing* that the period from post–World War II to the 1970s was a time of easy money, and healthcare costs continued to increase unchecked. Nonetheless, by the 1980s, Gavin (1980–1981, 5) noted succinctly, "Times have changed."

His voice was prophetic. Times have changed. Even with cost containment measures, healthcare costs continue to rise. As shown in Exhibit 2.1, the share of gross domestic product—the monetary value of all goods and services produced annually in the United States—attributable to expenditures on healthcare has steadily increased.

Healthcare providers have taken into account marketing as a method to help address what changes they should make to survive and thrive. Consider the changing trend regarding length of stay in a hospital. In 1970, the median length of stay for childbirth was four days. By 1992, the median had dropped to two days (CDC 1995). As Clarke (1978) suggested, the general decline in patient days (length of stay in a hospital) affected hospitals' income. Consequently, hospital administrators thought about further diversifying their services and became more open to marketing efforts in healthcare. For example,

1970	1980	1990	2000	2008
7.1%	9.0%	12.2%	13.4%	16.0%

Source: OECD (2010).

EXHIBIT 2.1

Total Expenditures on Health as a Share of Gross Domestic Product in the United States

with shorter inpatient hospital stays, attention turned to outpatient services. Organizations began to offer outpatient surgery, emphasizing the amenities they provided for family members waiting for a patient undergoing a procedure.

One prominent example was the "Blue Blazer" campaign started by a regional medical center in the 1970s. The hospital hired college students who were interested in working in medicine (pre-pharmacy, premed, pre–allied health, and pre-nursing). They wore blue blazers and helped make patients' family members comfortable at the surgery center. They parked cars so that family members could enter the center immediately rather than navigate the parking garage; accompanied them to waiting areas; and brought coffee, tea, and pastries for them to enjoy while the patient was in surgery. Family members knew that those wearing a blue blazer were at their service. While the Blue Blazers could not answer medical questions, they were willing and eager to listen to family members, fetch needed items, and attend to them in general. A pamphlet describing this service was displayed in the waiting rooms of local physicians' offices; billboards featuring the young, healthy-looking Blue Blazers were posted at key traffic points in the surrounding area; and the students were interviewed on a local television midday talk show to promote the service.

The result was positive. The regional medical center was operating at capacity within four months of launching the Blue Blazer campaign and increased its outpatient operations shortly thereafter. Drawn in by the service, customers (in this instance, patients and their family members) began to request that surgeries be performed at the regional medical center instead of elsewhere.

Let's consider the campaign in detail via a healthcare marketing lens. The regional medical center's administrators became aware that changing healthcare policy was negatively affecting the way they usually earned their money. With the decline in the length of inpatient hospital stays, they turned their attention to outpatient services. First, the administrators needed to determine their **target market**—the segment of the population they wanted to attract and engage. In this case, the target market was patients' family members. Second, they needed to determine what services and actions would attract this target market to the regional medical center for outpatient surgery. The regional medical center was in an urban environment, with parking mainly at a garage two blocks away from the outpatient center. Family members had been driving to the center to drop off patients at the entrance and then leaving to find a parking space. Providing a parking service—at no additional charge—was meeting a need. It was a service that had value. Third, the administrators needed to spread awareness of the Blue Blazer service. They did so in three ways—written communication in pamphlets placed in physicians' waiting rooms, visual communication via billboard placement, and oral and visual communication via the talk show interview. Finally, the medical center had to deliver the services it was promoting.

target market
the segment of a population a provider wants to attract and engage

Changing Consumer Expectations

The US public health system has published *Healthy People* objectives since 1991. *Healthy People 2000, Healthy People 2010*, and *Healthy People 2020* all focus on ten-year goals directed toward its vision: a society in which all people live long, healthy lives (HHS 2012). By educating consumers about their health and focusing on wellness and prevention, the initiative aims to bring about a healthier, more informed population. Not only do people learn how to be healthier and prevent illnesses; their efforts also reduce their healthcare costs and those of their payer, if they have access to insurance (e.g., employer-provided health insurance via organizations such as Blue Cross/Blue Shield, or the government—Medicare for Americans aged 65 or older, Medicaid for low-income Americans, and TRICARE for veterans). The return has been impressive. For instance, Johnson & Johnson's wellness programs, designed to educate Johnson & Johnson's employees about their health and focused on wellness and prevention, are in alignment with what *Healthy People* initiatives strive to do. Johnson & Johnson's programs have saved the company about $250 million in healthcare expenditures—roughly $2.71 for every dollar spent by the company (Berry, Mirabito, and Baun 2010). Clearly, education of healthcare consumers translates into positive outcomes cost-wise (reduction of costs) as well as health-wise (healthier consumers).

The initiative has also spurred an interest among consumers to be more involved in their healthcare rather than merely a patient. Past research found that healthcare consumers in Europe shared this interest (Tritter et al. 2010). US patients also have established expectations about their care experience. For instance, patients want healthcare providers to communicate with them and treat them with courtesy and respect (Liu et al. 2008; Otani, Herrmann, and Kurz 2011) and encourage them to participate in decision making about their care (Squires 2012). Patients also expect to be seen promptly, within 30 minutes of their scheduled appointment time (Hill and Joonas 2005).

Changing Attitudes Regarding the Stigma of Marketing by the Healthcare Profession

The first formal meeting on marketing sponsored by the American Hospital Association in 1977 marked the beginning of the field of healthcare marketing (MacStravic 1990). The first book on marketing in healthcare also was published that year (MacStravic 1977). The entrance of marketing into the healthcare arena was by no means smooth, quick, or readily embraced. It was resisted by healthcare providers and administrators and stigmatized as a practice that had no place in the field.

Sociologist Erving Goffman (1963) defined **stigma** as a discredited attribute. Consequently, those who have the attribute are looked upon negatively. For example, consider the stigma attached to people with mental illness. Because their illness is not

stigma
a discredited attribute

immediately perceptible and their behavior makes some people uncomfortable, those with mental illness may be stigmatized and ostracized.

Marketing, of course, is not mental illness, and the stigma attached to it is not directed toward individuals. However, the field of marketing is typically associated with the selling of some product, and selling was considered to be inappropriate for the healthcare profession (Robinson and Cooper 1980–1981). Its perceived inappropriateness arose from the theme that marketing clashed with tradition in the healthcare profession, which centered on the "intimate relationship" between physicians and patients (Cebrzynski 1985, 1). Moreover, some healthcare professionals viewed marketing as "frivolous and unnecessary and, at the worst, it was unethical" (Bryan and Gauff 1986, 11).

The American Medical Association (AMA) code of ethics of 1847 described advertising (a part of marketing) as "the ordinary practices of empirics, highly reprehensible in a regular physician" (Leake 1975, 224, as cited in Rizzo and Zeckhauser 1990, 480). Professors Rizzo (economics and preventive medicine) and Zeckhauser (political economy) (1990) offered a history of restrictions on physician advertising. In brief, the Federal Trade Commission (FTC) brought a complaint against the AMA in 1975 because the AMA did not allow physicians to advertise. The AMA responded in 1976, stating it was opposed to solicitation (an attempt to gain patients), not advertising (an avenue to informing). The clarification did not appease the FTC, and by 1982, the courts had sided with the FTC. Professionals, including physicians, could advertise—and they did, as evidenced by the introductory statement of a 2012 article on hospital advertising: "Nowadays, marketing has become a prominent function for healthcare organizations" (Nanda, Telang, and Bhatt 2012, 28).

MARKETING/PUBLIC RELATIONS DEPARTMENTS

Marketing in healthcare is no longer stigmatized as long as the marketing message is true, ethical, and not deceptive. Hospitals and clinics have departments and units dedicated to marketing activities. The names of these units vary among organizations. For example, one hospital might employ marketing personnel in its "marketing and public affairs office," another hospital might have an "office of marketing and public relations," and yet another might have a "department of business development, marketing, and community relations."

public relations
communicating information about an organization to the public to build understanding and support

The term **public relations**, however, is different from the term *healthcare marketing*. According to the Merriam-Webster online dictionary, *public relations* refers to "the business of inducing the public to have understanding for and goodwill toward a person, firm, or institution." Public relations in healthcare centers on conveying information from the healthcare organization to patients, physicians, the public, and payers. Healthcare marketing is broader than healthcare public relations. In addition to communicating information, healthcare marketing is about creating and delivering healthcare offerings.

In many healthcare settings, the appointment of public relations officers predated the introduction of marketing officers. The public relations office assumed marketing tasks, and the name of the office remained. Whatever the departments are called, their missions are the same: They create, communicate, and deliver offerings that have value for healthcare patients, physicians, the public, and payers.

HEALTHCARE "CUSTOMERS"

At the core of this text is the recognition that **healthcare customers** are more than one entity. They include patients, physicians, the public, and payers. Patients use services provided by clinics, hospitals, and physician practices. Physicians are customers of hospitals and clinics, not because they use services but because they refer their patients to hospitals and clinics. If physicians' needs are not met, they may refer their patients elsewhere.

healthcare customers patients, physicians, the public, and payers

The public is a customer because the community has a responsibility to protect the health of its residents, and decisions made by hospitals, for example, impact the public. Should a hospital build a new cardiovascular center? Purchase the latest technological robot for heart surgery? Hold smoking cessation classes? Support breast cancer awareness activities? Answers to such questions affect the public's ability to access healthcare and learn about wellness and prevention. They also affect healthcare providers' ability to serve the public.

Last, but not least, payers also are customers. Payers include private insurance companies (e.g., Blue Cross/Blue Shield), the government (i.e., Medicare for older Americans, Medicaid for low-income Americans, and TRICARE for veterans), and self-payers (i.e., individuals who pay out of pocket). Persons who work in marketing/public relations/community relations departments may not be at the table negotiating reimbursement with third-party payers or phoning patients to remind them to pay the remainder of their bill, but nonetheless, payers provide the money hospitals, clinics, and physician practices need to continue to conduct business and thus are customers, too.

Healthcare marketers work with all four entities to plan, implement, and evaluate healthcare initiatives, practices, and programs. They want patients, physicians, the public, and payers to think about their healthcare facility when contemplating health and healthcare.

CHAPTER QUESTIONS

1. Differentiate between the terms *public relations* and *healthcare marketing*. Look at five hospital websites. What do they name the department engaged in healthcare marketing? What is the relationship between public relations and healthcare marketing in US hospitals?
2. Provide examples of situations in which patients, physicians, the public, and payers are healthcare customers.
3. Explain why healthcare marketers became more valuable to healthcare organizations as consumer expectations changed.

1. *We aren't causing people to experience conditions—we are allowing them to experience them.*

    Mayo Clinic provides a grand piano in its atrium for anyone to play. This healthscape brings people together to laugh and share stories. Access the blog post "Mayo Clinic Music Fun" at http://sharing.mayoclinic.org/2009/04/07/mayo-clinic-music-fun/, and read about the impromptu and planned events that have occurred around the piano. Check out some of the videos and links, and scroll down to read some of the comments people have made about the post. Also peruse some of the pages hyperlinked at the end of the second column (e.g., News Blog, Online Health Community). Write a few paragraphs in which you

    ➤ explain why the healthscape is marketing for Mayo Clinic,

    ➤ identify the customers served by the atrium and the events that occur around the piano, and

    ➤ elaborate how the atrium and these events offer value to Mayo Clinic's customers.

    Next, choose one of the pages you perused and answer the following questions:

    ➤ How does it serve as marketing for Mayo Clinic?

    ➤ What customers does it serve?

    ➤ How does it offer value to customers?

2. *The public is a customer, too.*

    Consider the statement that the public is a healthcare customer. Go to the website of your local hospital (if you have more than one local hospital, select one of them), and see if it features a link to wellness and prevention services. If it does not, go to the website of another hospital in your region. Explain why this linked site is a marketing effort to educate the public about wellness and prevention as well as a marketing effort on behalf of the hospital. In your explanation, identify and consider other customers (patients, physicians, and/or payers) the site addresses. Finally, explain how the linked site offers value to the customer.

REFERENCES

American Marketing Association (AMA). 2007. "About AMA: Definition of Marketing." www.marketingpower.com/AboutAMA/Pages/DefinitionofMarketing.aspx.

Altringer, B. 2010. "The Emotional Experience of Patient Care: A Case for Innovation in Health Care Design." *Journal of Health Services Research & Policy* 15 (3): 174–77.

Berry, L. L., A. M. Mirabito, and W. B. Baun. 2010. "What's the Hard Return on Employee Wellness Programs?" *Harvard Business Review* 88 (12): 104–12.

Bitner, M. J. 1992. "Servicescapes: The Impact of Physical Surroundings on Customers and Employees." *Journal of Marketing* 56 (2): 57–71.

Bryan, G. O., and J. F. Gauff Jr. 1986. "Marketing 'Health Care Marketing.'" *Health Marketing Quarterly* 3 (4): 11–23.

Cebrzynski, G. 1985. "Marketing, Tradition Clash in Health Care." *Marketing News* 19 (23): 1–30.

Centers for Disease Control and Prevention (CDC). 1995. "Trends in Length of Stay for Hospital Deliveries—United States, 1970–1992." *MMWR Weekly* 44 (17): 335–37.

Clarke, R. N. 1978. "Marketing Health Care: Problems in Implementation." *Health Care Management Review* 3 (1): 21–27.

Dodson, D. C. 1985. "Health Care Marketing: Advancements but No Cigar." *Health Marketing Quarterly* 2 (4): 13–23.

Dunlap, B. J., and D. C. Dodson. 1980–1981. "From the Editors." *Journal of Health Care Marketing* 1 (1): 4.

Fottler, M. D., R. C. Ford, V. Roberts, and E. W. Ford. 2000. "Creating a Healing Environment: The Importance of the Service Setting in the New Consumer-Oriented Healthcare System." *Journal of Healthcare Management* 45 (2): 91–106.

Gavin, M. 1980–1981. "A Survival Manual for Health Care Providers in the Competitive Marketplace." *Journal of Health Care Marketing* 1 (1): 5–6.

Goffman, E. 1963. *Stigma: Notes on the Management of Spoiled Identity*. London: Penguin.

Hill, C. J., and K. Joonas. 2005. "The Impact of Unacceptable Wait Time on Health Care Patients' Attitudes and Actions." *Health Marketing Quarterly* 23 (2): 69–87.

Hume, J. 2009. "A Bite of Life." Posted April 23. http://sharing.mayoclinic.org/2009/04/23/a-bite-of-life/.

Kotler, P. 1975. *Marketing for Nonprofit Organizations*. Englewood Cliffs, NJ: Prentice-Hall.

Kotler, P., and S. J. Levy. 1969. "Broadening the Concept of Marketing." *Journal of Marketing* 33 (1): 10–15.

Leake, C. D. (ed.) 1975. *Percival's Medical Ethics*, reprint edition. Huntington, NY: Robert E. Krieger Publishing Company.

Liu, S. S., E. Amendah, E. C. Chang, and L. K. Pei. 2008. "Satisfaction and Value: A Meta-Analysis in the Healthcare Context." *Health Marketing Quarterly* 23 (4): 49–73.

MacStravic, R. E. 1990. "The End of Health Care Marketing?" *Health Marketing Quarterly* 7 (1-2): 3–7.

———. 1977. *Marketing Health Care*. Gaithersburg, MD: Aspen.

Nanda, S., A. Telang, and G. Bhatt. 2012. "Hospital Advertising: A Literature Review." *International Journal of Healthcare Management* 5 (1): 28–31.

Organisation for Economic Co-operation and Development (OECD). 2010. "OECD Health Data: Health Expenditure and Financing." *OECD Health Statistics* (database). DOI: 10.1787/data-00350-en.

Otani, K., P. A. Herrmann, and R. S. Kurz. 2011. "Improving Patient Satisfaction in Hospital Care Settings." *Health Services Management Research* 24 (4): 163–69.

Rizzo, J. A., and R. J. Zeckhauser. 1990. "Advertising and Entry: The Case of Physician Services." *Journal of Political Economy* 98 (3): 476–500.

Robinson, L. M., and P. D. Cooper. 1980–1981. "Roadblocks to Hospital Marketing." *Journal of Health Care Marketing* 1 (1): 18–24.

Squires, S. 2012. "Patient Satisfaction: How to Get It and How to Keep It." *Nursing Management* 43 (4): 26–32.

Tritter, J., M. Koivusalo, E. Ollila, and P. Dorfman. 2010. *Globalisation, Markets and Healthcare Policy: Redrawing the Patient as Consumer.* New York: Routledge.

US Department of Health and Human Services (HHS). 2012. "About Healthy People." www.healthypeople.gov/2020/about/default.aspx.

Winston, W. J. 1986. "The Evolution of Hospital Marketing." *Journal of Hospital Marketing* 1 (1-2): 19–28.

CHAPTER 3

STRATEGY AND HEALTHCARE MARKETING

After studying this chapter, you will be able to

➤ describe the importance of mission, vision, and goals in healthcare organizations and their relationship to—and interaction with—marketing; and

➤ discuss the relationship between marketing and research in the development of sound organizational strategy.

CASE STUDY: MISSION, VISION, AND GOALS AT SUNNY DAY

The new administrator of the Sunny Day skilled nursing facility (SNF) began his first staff meeting with these words:

> Long-term care is vastly misunderstood. People don't really understand it unless they work in a nursing home—and even then, lots of nursing home employees still don't really understand it. Even our residents and their families don't get it. Sunny Day is part of this great misconception, and it is going to stop. Starting today, we are going to create and implement a new mission, a new vision, and new goals, and they are going to guide everything we do every moment of every day. Everyone in this town is going to know our mission, vision, and goals and will be able to see how we live up to them. I'm charging you, Mark, as director of marketing, to lead this endeavor. Put together your team. I want to see results by next month's staff meeting.

Mark Krainz was not exactly happy to have been assigned this task. He had earned his degree in healthcare administration, so he was familiar with the concept and importance of mission, vision, and goals (MVG), but he thought they were the responsibility of top management. He had no idea what marketing had to do with MVG. Despite his initial misgivings about the assignment, he began reviewing Sunny Day's long-standing MVG statements:

> Sunny Day Nursing Home exists to provide the finest and highest quality of care to its patients. We strive to be leaders in the field of long-term care, and we do so by employing only the best caregivers and using only the newest and best treatments and procedures. We are proud to be a government-accredited skilled nursing facility.

All those things were certainly true about Sunny Day, but Mark wanted to see what other nursing homes' MVGs looked like. Lots of the local SNFs didn't even have websites, and when he called and asked them to send their MVGs, many SNFs were hesitant, to the point of refusing to share this information with him. When he finally received a few MVGs from other SNFs, he noticed that they all said pretty much the same thing.

Mark knew without a doubt that Sunny Day had the best reputation and provided the best care in town. He knew that he and his team could build better MVG statements for Sunny Day, and he was eager to start working on them. Now, who should be on his MVG team?

ORGANIZATIONAL STRATEGY AND HEALTHCARE MARKETING

strategy
an overarching plan designed to achieve a goal

tactics
the specific actions taken to achieve a goal

objectives
long-term performance and outcome goals

The idea of **strategy**—a plan designed to achieve a goal—originated in the military. Strategy is often confused with **tactics**, which are the specific actions taken to achieve a goal. Strategy is also often confused with objectives. **Objectives** are long-term performance and outcome goals. Strategy is more comprehensive than tactics and objectives; it is an overarching plan. Strategic planning can and should occur in an organization at many levels. For example, marketing strategy is an overarching plan that enables an organization to concentrate its limited resources on its greatest opportunities to increase sales, attain its goals, and sustain a competitive advantage (Baker 2008, 3). It is informed by careful analysis of the organization's internal and external environments by the organization's marketing research process. Finally, strategies at all organizational levels must align with and support the organization's mission, vision, and values. This chapter begins with a discussion of mission, vision, and values in healthcare organizations and concludes with an explanation of the important role that healthcare marketing plays in achieving an organization's mission and vision and living its values.

MISSION AND VISION

mission statement
the embodiment and self-image of an organization; a declaration that expresses an organization's highest goals and provides strategic direction

An organization's **mission statement** is essential to its ongoing success (Bart and Tabone 1998). At the least, an organization's mission statement should help to distinguish it from other organizations (Griffith 1988). At its best, a mission statement is the embodiment and self-image of an organization. The mission expresses the highest goals of an organization and provides strategic direction (Wiggins, Hatzenbuehler, and Peterson 2008). An organization without a clear, achievable mission is like a traveler without a road map. You seem to be making good time, but you don't really know where you are going to end up.

In today's increasingly competitive healthcare industry, it is imperative that mission-driven healthcare organizations—whether hospitals, physician practices, long-term care facilities, durable medical equipment distributors, or pharmaceutical companies—be able to achieve and maintain a clear, identifiable reputation; name recognition; and competitive advantage. What, if anything, distinguishes one hospital from all other hospitals, one pharmaceutical firm from another, or one group of physicians from any other group of physicians? For many decades, this need to set one's organization apart from all other organizations of a similar nature was greatly hampered by the healthcare industry's misunderstanding of—and disdain for—marketing. Indeed, a 2005 study of hospital mission statements found that nearly all contained similar language and claims regarding their commitment to the provision of high-quality care (Bolon 2005). In a 2008 study, researchers searched a random sample of hospital mission statements for key words associated with interest in and commitment to education and found that the missions of 21 of the 81 (26 percent) teaching hospitals examined made no reference to teaching or education. More than 25 percent of teaching hospitals' missions were indistinguishable from nonteaching hospitals' missions (Wiggins, Hatzenbuehler, and Peterson 2008).

Certainly all healthcare organizations and providers are committed to providing quality care, but when their mission statements are homogenized and interchangeable, they cannot build a unique reputation or communicate a competitive advantage. Thus, if an organization's strategies must align with and actively support its overarching mission, and if its mission statement is indistinguishable from the missions of other healthcare organizations, how can marketing strategy adequately and ethically steer the organization's limited resources to the most appropriate opportunities for attaining and sustaining competitive advantage and achieving its mission?

An organization's **vision statement** is similar to its mission, but it extends beyond what the organization is into the realm of what the organization wants to be. An organization's vision is its ideal future state. It is the best that an organization can aspire to be. It describes the direction an organization wants to take and the desired end result of that journey (McConnell 2007). Put another way, if an organization were a person, what would it see when it closes its eyes and dreams? Healthcare organizations' visions can be inspiring and, perhaps, audacious. Consider, for example, the vision of a small community hospital in southern Idaho to "be a standard of excellence and cooperation in making Mountain Valley the healthiest place in America" (McGinnis et al. 2003). Seeing itself as the healthiest place in America certainly is an audacious dream, but it is a worthy vision to work toward.

It is not marketers' place or responsibility to badger their organization into recrafting and rewriting its mission and vision statements, although from a marketing point of view it might be a useful and productive endeavor. However, whether or not an organization's mission is bland and similar to those of other organizations of its kind, and whether or not the organization's vision is exciting, specific, and dynamic, it is the responsibility of the marketer to dig deeper into the statements and examine the organization's values.

vision statement
a declaration of an organization's ideal future state, the direction an organization wants to take to get there, and the desired end result

ORGANIZATIONAL VALUES

There is a lot of talk in healthcare about values. **Organizational values** are standards that govern the behavior of individuals in an organization. In an enterprise that encompasses almost innumerable professions, patients, providers, and customers, one needs to understand that each of these constituencies, as a group and as individuals, has its own value system. Without a common understanding and acceptance of established values, healthcare organizations would have to conduct business and deliver care while immersed in a veritable sea of opposing, contradictory, overlapping, and clashing values.

Values can be very personal and deeply held. In an industry in which each profession has its own code of ethics and patients and consumers have vastly diverse ethnicities,

organizational values
standards that govern the behavior of individuals in an organization

religions, backgrounds, and cultures, it is imperative that health organizations be clear, internally and externally, about the values on which they stand. In addition, healthcare leaders must understand that simply writing or posting a code of values does not mean that the people in their organization will actually embrace and live those values. Thus, it behooves healthcare organizations to become perfectly transparent value-wise as they strive to achieve their mission and fulfill their vision. The Teal Trust, a former leadership organization most known for its leadership style indicator, suggested that the following five activities encourage people to uphold behavioral norms that support the achievement of their organization's mission and vision:

1. Communicate values clearly and constantly both within and outside of the organization. Everyone inside and outside the organization knows what you represent.

2. Enroll new members of the organization in the culture of values immediately. Value-focused information and indoctrination should start with the selection process.

3. Revisit and refresh your values periodically. Healthcare is constantly changing; you must ensure that your organizational values have kept pace.

4. Confront contradictory behavior. Provide feedback to those who do not live the organization's values.

5. Periodically solicit feedback. Ask people, both inside and outside the organization, what they believe the organization's values are.

Clarity of values and a mission and vision that clearly delineate and set the organization apart from others of its kind are the lenses through which marketing can look to understand and align itself with the organization's internal and external environments.

HEALTHCARE SUCCESS AND MARKETING RESEARCH

Healthcare marketing is driven by the need for current and accurate information crucial to achieving an organization's mission and vision. Strong marketing research guides healthcare organizations to make sound decisions in all areas (Fell and Shepherd 2008, 1):

Good market research defines areas of concern for a healthcare organization, helps frame strategic decisions, and connects the management team with its customers and stakeholders . . . . If making good business decisions is the key to market growth and sustainability in healthcare, then market research should be considered a critical element in that decision-making process.

Two fundamental conditions in the healthcare industry are constant change and increasing competition. For most of the twentieth century, healthcare was internally focused, paying attention primarily to the needs of physicians, hospitals, and payers. The assumption was that when the needs of these three groups were met, the needs of patients also were met.

A healthcare organization's survival now depends on having a clear understanding of both its internal and external environments. Furthermore, a successful healthcare organization differentiates itself—separates itself from the pack, as it were—not only to attract patients but also to recruit and retain high-quality employees. No longer is a hospital just a hospital; no longer is a physician practice just a group of doctors that might as well be any group of doctors. Healthcare organizations need to understand, nurture, and trumpet their distinct competencies.

Healthcare organizations must be **consciously competent**—no luck or accident is involved. They need to know what works, with whom it works, and why it works. In addition, a successful organization understands that healthcare provides two kinds of value: visible and invisible. In this sense, value does not refer to the cultural standards of behavior discussed earlier. This time, value refers to the economic concept of worth, of cost versus benefit. **Visible value** is value that a customer can see. **Invisible value** is value that a producer builds into its product (Berkowitz 2011, 53). Both are fundamental to aligning an organization's marketing efforts with its mission, vision, and values.

When conducting market research, the healthcare marketer needs to determine what customers/patients need and desire. What will make their experience with the healthcare organization memorable and make them want to return? Interestingly, it is not always what marketers think it will be. Internally, organizations know they add value by using electronic medical records, credentialing caregivers, and providing continuing education for all staff—but most patients don't care about those things. Patients that do care about these features assume they are givens; their value is invisible. Patients want high-quality care, compassion, respect, and convenience—all visible values. Only by deeply understanding their organization's patients, customers, markets, and internal and external environments can marketers support and align their efforts with its mission, vision, and values.

consciously competent
knowing what works,
with whom it works,
and why it works

visible value
value that a customer
can see

invisible value
value that a producer
builds into its product

MARKETING THAT SUPPORTS THE MISSION

Healthcare organizations need to be both mission based and market driven; the two concepts are intertwined. Mission-based, market-driven organizations (Brinckerhoff 2010, 17–18)

◆   understand their markets;

◆   treat everyone like a customer;

◆ include everyone on the marketing team;

◆ ask, ask, ask, and then listen;

◆ innovate constantly;

◆ promote and protect their brand; and

◆ use every communication medium available.

These characteristics are not as straightforward in healthcare as they are in other industries. For example, healthcare markets comprise not only customers, consumers, and patients. They also include insurance companies; equipment and technology interests; and a huge assortment of health professionals, from physicians and nurses to accountants, lawyers, suppliers, and vendors. In an industry that is often uncomfortable using the word *customer*, how does an organization treat everyone as such? How can it treat physicians as customers? Healthcare professionals traditionally think of themselves by discipline, not by employer. A nurse is a nurse who happens to work at St. Rita Hospital, not an employee of St. Rita who happens to be a nurse. And almost universally, health professionals don't see themselves as marketers in any sense of the word.

principal–agent relationship
the principal (patient) gives consent for the agent (caregiver) to have the authority and power to make appropriate decisions on her or his behalf

The **principal–agent relationship** may no longer rule supreme in today's healthcare industry, but it still exists: The principal (patient) gives consent for the agent (caregiver) to have the authority and power to make appropriate decisions on her or his behalf (Berkowitz 2011, 52). It is assumed that patients rarely understand their own healthcare wants and needs, and thus the idea of ask, ask, ask, and then listen may be a foreign and perhaps frightening concept for caregivers. After all, regardless of what patients may think they want or need, providers have care protocols, regulations, and professional standards they must uphold.

In a world where most hospital mission statements are incredibly similar, what is a hospital's brand? Does the word *brand* even have meaning in healthcare? These questions are rhetorical, of course, and are addressed in later sections of this book. The point here is that market-driven concepts such as those presented in these questions must be at the core of a mission-driven organization, and healthcare organizations present unique challenges in this respect.

In particular, it is important to understand that marketing in healthcare is far more than just advertising or attracting patients and customers to a facility. Some experts argue that marketing has evolved through three stages. Marketing 1.0 was product-centric and focused on sales, and Marketing 2.0 was focused on corporate positioning and satisfying and retaining customers. Marketing 3.0 emphasizes that consumers are no longer isolated individuals; they are empowered and connected via any number of media channels, and their knowledge and behavior change organizations and products (Kotler, Kartajaya, and

Setiawan 2010). Consider the urban clothing store Gap. When Gap made minor changes to its original logo, the negative customer outcry via social media was so strong that Gap quickly returned to using the original (Parr 2010). Another example is the Susan G. Komen Foundation's decision to change its funding of Planned Parenthood. Like Gap's experience, the strong negative pressure exerted through social media caused the foundation to reverse its funding decision (CNN Wire Staff 2012). The cautionary tale and lesson learned are that any organization that does not know its environments and markets, does not listen to its customers and stakeholders, and acts as if its business decisions are best made in the vacuum of the corporate offices often suffers and finds itself retrenching.

Peter Drucker (1989), who is often called the father of modern management, said that successful businesses don't start their planning with financials; they start by defining their mission, and performing their mission brings financial returns. Thus, the understanding of markets and customers garnered through marketing research is the foundation on which mission-driven, mission-achieving organizations are built.

CHAPTER QUESTIONS

1. Differentiate among these terms: *strategy, tactics,* and *objectives*; and *mission, vision,* and *values.*
2. Provide a healthcare example for each of the Teal Trust's five behavioral norms that help an organization achieve its mission and vision.
3. What is the relationship between marketing and mission achievement?

CHAPTER EXERCISES

1. *We're on a mission*

    Access a website for each of the following types of organizations, and find their mission/vision/values statements.

    ➤ University hospital

    ➤ Hospital/healthcare system

    ➤ Not-for-profit community hospital

    ➤ Ambulatory surgery center

    ➤ Skilled nursing facility

➤ Pharmaceutical company

➤ Mental/behavioral health center

Was it easy or difficult to find these organizations' mission/vision/values statements? What do their statements have in common? How do they differ? What conclusions can you draw about mission/vision/values statements in healthcare now that you have completed this exercise?

2. *Whose vision is it?*

You are the new assistant to the chief operating officer (COO) at a pediatric surgery group practice in Chicago. The practice has 15 physicians, 7 nurse practitioners/physician assistants, 27 nurses, and 10 support/administrative/office staff. You report directly to the COO, and the COO reports directly to the CEO, who is also the chief medical officer of the practice. The market for pediatrics in Chicago is very competitive, and your group practice has managed to make a slim profit every year in the ten years it has existed. The board of directors, which consists of all the physician owners, has charged the COO with creating and implementing a plan to ensure that the organization's values not only support the practice's mission and vision but also ensure a larger profit margin. The COO has passed this assignment down to you. Using the Teal Trust's five behavioral norms presented in this chapter in the section on organizational values, create an action plan for the COO to present at the next board meeting.

REFERENCES

Baker, M. 2008. *The Strategic Marketing Plan Audit*. Devon, UK: Cambridge Strategy Publications.

Bart, C. K., and J. C. Tabone. 1998. "Mission Statement Rationales and Organization Alignment in the Not-for-Profit Health Care Sector." *Health Care Management Review* 23 (4): 54–69.

Berkowitz, E. N. 2011. *Essentials of Health Care Marketing*, third edition. Sudbury, MA: Jones and Bartlett Learning.

Bolon, D. S. 2005. "Comparing Mission Statement Content in For-Profit and Not-for-Profit Hospitals: Does Mission Really Matter?" *Hospital Topics* 83 (4): 2–9.

Brinckerhoff, P. C. 2010. *Mission-Based Marketing*. Hoboken, NJ: John Wiley & Sons, Inc.

CNN Wire Staff. 2012. "Komen Foundation Reverses Funding Decision of Planned Parent-hood." Updated February 4. www.cnn.com/2012/02/03/politics/planned-parenthood-komen-foundation/index.html?_s=PM:POLITICS.

Drucker, P. F. 1989. "What Business Can Learn from Nonprofits." *Harvard Business Review* July. http://hbr.org/1989/07/what-business-can-learn-from-nonprofits/ar/1.

Griffith, J. R. 1988. "The Mission of the Well-Managed Community Hospital." *Michigan Hospitals* 24 (7): 43, 45–46.

Fell, D., and C. D. Shepherd. 2008. *A Marketer's Guide to Market Research*. Marblehead, MA: HCPro, Inc.

Kotler, P., H. Kartajaya, and I. Setiawan. 2010. *Marketing 3.0: From Products to Customers to the Human Spirit*. Hoboken, NJ: John Wiley and Sons, Inc.

McConnell, T. 2007. "What Is an Organization's Vision?" Posted March 20. http://voices.yahoo.com/what-organizations-vision-243081.html.

McGinnis, S., L. Pumphrey, K. Trimmer, and C. Wiggins. 2003. "Innovation in a Small, Rural Community Hospital: A Case Study Approach." Proceedings of the fourth annual Global Information Technology Management World Conference by Global Information Technology Management Association, Calgary, Alberta, June 8–10.

Parr, B. 2010. "Gap Reverts to Original Logo After Social Media Backlash." Published October 11. http://mashable.com/2010/10/11/gap-logo/.

Wiggins, C., L. Hatzenbuehler, and T. Peterson. 2008. "Hospital Missions and the Education of Our Future Health Care Workforce." *Journal of Allied Health* 37 (3): 132–36.

CHAPTER 4

ETHICS AND HEALTHCARE MARKETING

After studying this chapter, you will be able to

➤ explain the concept of healthcare marketing ethics,

➤ apply ethical frameworks to healthcare situations,

➤ create and defend a response to a situation while keeping ethical considerations in mind, and

➤ evaluate the role of the healthcare marketer in relation to ethical behavior and conduct.

CASE STUDY: EVERYDAY ETHICS AND PUBLIC RELATIONS IN HEALTHCARE

Mariana Bouvier walked swiftly to attend a special meeting; she had been called by the administrative assistant for the CEO, who had asked if Mariana could please "take a moment and come to the CEO's conference room now." Mariana had never been called to come to a meeting that was to take place "now," so she knew that it must be important.

Mariana was a public relations officer in the marketing department of Atlantic Medical University (AMU). The AMU campus included a teaching hospital and several clinics and employed more than 30,000 people. Mariana had graduated from Atlantic University two years previously with a degree in health administration. Having enjoyed her general business marketing and healthcare marketing classes, she completed an internship in the marketing department at AMU during her senior year.

The internship had required that she work 40 hours per week for six weeks, for a total of 240 hours. She had learned a lot about public relations, both inside and outside the hospital community, and about media communications, and she had written articles for *Atlantic Stars*, an internal monthly newsletter written for and about AMU employees, and for the quarterly community publication *Atlantic Community Healthcare*. She had also shadowed the marketing director, who was responsible for all media communications about AMU with the local television, radio, and newspaper reporters. When Mariana graduated, she was offered a position at AMU as a public relations officer. Her primary responsibilities were similar to the work she had done during her internship—overseeing the in-house and community publications. In addition, she was asked to take on the role of media contact formerly held by the marketing director. Mariana accepted the job. Over the next two years, her annual evaluations indicated that she had been doing outstanding work, and she loved her job! She was able to use her health administration skills and enjoyed working with her colleagues.

Mariana entered the CEO's conference room and noticed that she, her supervisor, and the marketing director had arrived first. Shortly thereafter, others entered, including the chief financial officer (CFO), the hospital's attorney, the chief information officer (CIO), the human resources director, and the administrator of AMU's SportsMed clinic. In her two years at AMU, Mariana's contact with the Atlantic SportsMed clinic had been minimal; she had written an article for *Atlantic Stars* on the clinic's three original physician owners and had fielded media questions a few months ago when a celebrity went to the clinic for care after breaking his hand while vacationing in the area. Mariana took notes while the clinic's administrator explained the reason for the meeting. "As you know," the administrator began, "Atlantic SportsMed is one of AMU's clinics. It seems that Medicare is investigating the clinic for fraudulent claims."

ATLANTIC SPORTSMED CLINIC'S HISTORY

Atlantic SportsMed was a clinic that specialized in orthopedics, podiatry, rehabilitation medicine, and pain management. The original physician owners of Atlantic SportsMed (Drs. Laroche, Chevalier, and Dupont) had sold the clinic to AMU five years previously. The contract between Atlantic SportsMed and AMU specified that these three physicians were to earn a salary of $200,000 each annually. If Atlantic SportsMed generated a profit, each physician would earn an additional 10 percent of the total profit. For example, if Atlantic SportsMed generated a profit of $500,000 annually, the three physicians would earn an additional $50,000 each. All of the other providers at the clinic—12 orthopedic physicians, a physiatrist, a pain management physician, and three podiatrists—earned only a salary. The clinic's mid-level providers—eight physical therapists, three occupational therapists, and seven nurses—and the administrative team of three clinic managers, two coders/billers, and six receptionists earned only a salary as well.

The clinic was busy. The physicians and staff had developed excellent provider–patient relationships. Its patients were returning customers, and word-of-mouth promotion drew new customers. Atlantic SportsMed was one of the highest income producers for AMU.

Recently, one of the coders/billers reported Atlantic SportsMed to the Medicare Fraud Control Units, and Medicare notified AMU that it was investigating the clinic; Drs. Laroche, Chevalier, and Dupont; and AMU and was auditing the clinic's accounts.

The administrator continued to explain the situation to Mariana and the others in the conference room. "Five hundred and eighty-nine geriatric patients—older than 65 and insured by Medicare—have been longtime patients at SportsMed. Over the past year, each has visited at least twice per month on average, and each visit included one 15-minute session of therapy during which the patient threw and caught a ball with a physical therapist to manipulate and increase the strength and range of motion of the patient's hands. The coding for this treatment is CPT 97530. Medicare approved payment of this treatment as long as the patient was improving. In the medical records of all 589 patients, physicians noted that the patients were improving. However, in 447 of these same records, physical therapists indicated that the patients were not improving. The coder questioned the submission of claims for this treatment when patients' records indicated that they were not improving, but she was told to bill Medicare for the treatments anyway. Concerned, she reported the incident to the Medicare Fraud Control Units. The investigation revealed that the SportsMed clinic received $57.20 from Medicare for each treatment. Over the course of a year, the Medicare reimbursement per patient was $57.20 × 24 = $1,372.80 because, as I stated earlier, each patient was treated an average of two times per month over the past 12 months. Thus, for the 447 patients whose records indicated they were *not improving*, Medicare reimbursed the clinic a total of $613,641.60."

Mariana's cell phone vibrated, and she looked down to read the text message that had just arrived. It was from the local television reporter, who had typed, "Hi Mariana. Heard about SportsMed clinic. Want to make a comment? Call me."

HEALTHCARE MARKETING ETHICS CONSIDERED

Healthcare ethics refers to moral standards of clinical and administrative conduct that affect healthcare stakeholders. **Stakeholders** are people, groups, and organizations that "hold a stake" in an enterprise and are affected by the conduct of people in that enterprise. In the case study, stakeholders included the patients who underwent the hand therapy, the coder who was told to bill for the treatment, other salaried providers and staff at the SportsMed clinic, the three physicians who had previously owned the clinic, the clinic's leadership team, the employees of AMU, AMU itself, and the general public.

In everyday life, individuals' personal moral codes guide their behaviors and actions. At times, people must seriously consider whether actions they are contemplating violate those codes. Exhibit 4.1 categorizes example behaviors/actions in one of four quadrants to illustrate their legal/ethical status. (While Exhibit 4.1 is substantively in the public domain, it is possibly based on ethics professor and management consultant Verne Henderson's (1982) concentric circle model, which illustrates how ethics may be conceptualized in business.) Behaviors/actions may be unethical and illegal, ethical and legal, unethical but legal, or ethical but illegal. Stealing drugs is wrong; providing a patient with expert care is right. However, controversial topics, such as assisted suicide and expediting a celebrity's organ transplant, provoke debate. Whether these latter two examples are right or wrong is not as clear.

Beginning with the Hippocratic Oath, healthcare is governed by ethical codes of clinical conduct. Each of the clinical professions has a specific **professional code of ethics** that spells out ethical/professional standards of conduct/behavior for its members. Examples include

- ◆ the American Medical Association's (AMA) Code of Medical Ethics for physicians (www.ama-assn.org), and

- ◆ the American Physical Therapy Association's (APTA) Code of Ethics for the Physical Therapist (www.apta.org).

healthcare ethics
moral standards of clinical and administrative conduct that affect healthcare stakeholders

stakeholders
people, groups, and organizations that "hold a stake" in an enterprise and are affected by the conduct of people in that enterprise

professional code of ethics
ethical/professional standards of conduct/behavior for members of a profession

Action	Unethical	Ethical
Illegal	Stealing prescription drugs from a hospital's pharmacy	Assisted suicide (encourages debate)
Legal	Expediting a celebrity's organ transplant (encourages debate)	Expertly assisting patients who cannot get up from their hospital beds

EXHIBIT 4.1
Quadrants of Ethical/Legal Behavior

Administrative and managerial professionals in the healthcare environment also have specific professional codes of ethics. Coding and marketing professionals are two examples:

◆ For coders, the American Health Information Management Association (AHIMA) not only has a code of ethics but also outlines expectations for ethical decision making in the workplace (www.ahima.org). AHIMA's framework is reproduced in Exhibit 4.2. Moreover, AHIMA provides case studies to assist its members' ethical decision making in the workplace. The case studies illustrate work situations in which ethics had a role and show how the professional addressed the situation.

◆ For healthcare marketers, the American College of Healthcare Executives (ACHE) provides a code of ethics and a process to assist with ethical decision making (www.ache.org).

While AMA and APTA focus on clinical behaviors and AHIMA and ACHE center on administrative and managerial conduct, they share four fundamental ethical standards: justice, fidelity, beneficence, and autonomy (Beauchamp and Childress 2001). Think about the characters in the case study, and identify the courses of action they should take. What factors should Mariana keep in mind as she communicates with the reporter? What considerations do the standards of justice, fidelity, and beneficence require of her?

HEALTHCARE MARKETERS AND ETHICAL BEHAVIOR

justice
ensuring that people are treated fairly to bring about a fair outcome

The **justice** standard addresses the importance of properly and appropriately communicating the issue so that it is handled ethically and fairly. The philosopher John Rawls (1971) introduced the concept of *procedural justice* as the adoption of a fair procedure to bring about an equitable outcome. He illustrated his concept using a simple example of allocating slices of cake. If one person is told to cut a cake and let others choose their slices first, the person will cut equally sized slices so that he is assured an equal share (Rawls 1971, 84). Hence, a fair process effects a fair outcome. Healthcare marketers often make decisions in which fairness plays a role because they influence how stakeholders—employees (internal) and the general public (external)—are treated.

Along with a fair process, the manner in which employees are treated in interactions affects employees' behavior (Dessler 2009). *Interactional justice* refers to how people are treated (interpersonal justice) and how much information is given to them (informational justice). If she follows this standard, Mariana will consider what she shares with the local television reporter and be mindful of her need to be fair to AMU employees.

EXHIBIT 4.2
AHIMA Standards
of Ethical Coding

Coding professionals should:

1. Apply accurate, complete, and consistent coding practices for the production of high-quality healthcare data.
2. Report all healthcare data elements (e.g., diagnosis and procedure codes, present on admission indicator, discharge status) required for external reporting purposes (e.g., reimbursement and other administrative uses, population health, quality and patient safety measurement, and research) completely and accurately, in accordance with regulatory and documentation standards and requirements and applicable official coding conventions, rules, and guidelines.
3. Assign and report only the codes and data that are clearly and consistently supported by health record documentation in accordance with applicable code set and abstraction conventions, rules, and guidelines.
4. Query provider (physician or other qualified healthcare practitioner) for clarification and additional documentation prior to code assignment when there is conflicting, incomplete, or ambiguous information in the health record regarding a significant reportable condition or procedure or other reportable data element dependent on health record documentation (e.g., present on admission indicator).
5. Refuse to change reported codes or the narratives of codes so that meanings are misrepresented.
6. Refuse to participate in or support coding or documentation practices intended to inappropriately increase payment, qualify for insurance policy coverage, or skew data by means that do not comply with federal and state statutes, regulations and official rules and guidelines.
7. Facilitate interdisciplinary collaboration in situations supporting proper coding practices.
8. Advance coding knowledge and practice through continuing education.
9. Refuse to participate in or conceal unethical coding or abstraction practices or procedures.
10. Protect the confidentiality of the health record at all times and refuse to access protected health information not required for coding-related activities (examples of coding-related activities include completion of code assignment, other health record data abstraction, coding audits, and educational purposes).
11. Demonstrate behavior that reflects integrity, shows a commitment to ethical and legal coding practices, and fosters trust in professional activities.

The **fidelity** standard is about loyalty and faithfulness to duty. With regard to this standard, Mariana's job is to ensure that her communications are accurate and true, but again, she must carefully consider AMU employees' rights as well. Additionally, authors Eva Winkler and Russell Gruen (2005, 109) elaborate on the fidelity standard to propose that organizational ethics include managers' responsibility to be compassionate regarding healthcare delivery, respectful to their employees, public spirited, and mindful of their organization's resources. This standard also extends to healthcare professionals as corporate citizens (Cellucci and Wiggins 2010, 27). They are loyal to their discipline and mindful of the environment and community in which they live.

The **beneficence** standard refers to the professional duty to benefit others. This principle is based on the Hippocratic Oath, which states that physicians must apply all measures required to benefit the sick and do no harm (Goldberg 1963).

The **autonomy** standard is based on the premise that people are able to make informed decisions that respect and consider the well-being of others. This principle was one of the foci of the *Belmont Report*, which included ethical principles and guidelines for the protection of human research subjects. The report was published in 1979 by the National Commission for the Protection of Human Subjects of Biomedical and Behavioral Research after controversial studies such as the Tuskegee syphilis experiment were made public and the ethical standing of such research was called into question.

HEALTHCARE MARKETERS AS CRITICAL THINKERS AND CREATIVE PROBLEM SOLVERS

The concepts that guide ethical behavior and decision making for healthcare professionals help them think critically and solve problems creatively. As AMU's public relations officer, Mariana has ethical frameworks she is obligated to consider as she fulfills her responsibilities. First and foremost, the problem must be defined correctly.

The ethical dilemma in the case study varies among the different characters. For the physicians at the clinic, the ethical principles pose potential conflicts. The physicians are to do no harm, respect patients' autonomy and rights, faithfully treat patients to heal their hands, and be honest. If Medicare denies payment for the treatment, patients probably will stop going to the clinic for therapy. If the patients stop going to the clinic and receiving hand therapy, the likelihood of any improvement is practically nil. Continued hand therapy may bring about some improvement. By noting in patients' records that they were improving, the physicians acted in accordance with the principles of fidelity and beneficence (their duty to heal) but possibly counter to the principle of autonomy (honesty).

The coder's dilemma points out the value of the ethical principles as well. The coder is responsible for coding practices and values accuracy in patients' information. The patients' records indicate contradictory information, and thus it does not appear to be accurate and true. Moreover, the coder, as a professional, has an obligation to act.

Mariana also must strike an ethical balance. Her position obligates her to give the reporter accurate and true information but also to adhere to the standards of procedural and informational justice to ensure that the clinic's employees are treated fairly.

When the coder discovered the inconsistencies in the patients' records, she may have asked herself whether she had addressed each AHIMA standard appropriately. For instance, the patients' records indicated contradictory information regarding improvement. She followed AHIMA standard #4 by asking the provider about the conflicting notes. However, she was told to bill Medicare for the treatments anyway and was not provided documentation to support such billing. The coder followed AHIMA standards when she subsequently reported her concerns about the inconsistent documentation in patients' records to Medicare.

Jacqueline Glover, professor in the Center for Bioethics and Humanities at University of Colorado Denver, offers an ethical decision-making process for health information managers dealing with challenging ethical problems. While specifically designed for health informatics professionals, these steps also apply to decision making by healthcare marketing administrators such as Mariana. Glover's (2006) process includes seven steps:

1. *What is the ethical question?* In the case study, Mariana learns that Medicare is investigating fraudulent practices. Because of her position in the marketing department of the hospital, her responsibility to be mindful of ethical standards is framed by her communications with the media. Thus, for Mariana, the ethical question is, what information is appropriate to share with the media?

2. *What are the facts?* The facts in the case study are twofold: those that are known and those that are being gathered. Mariana needs to be mindful that certain facts are known, Medicare is investigating the situation, and the patients' documentation is contradictory as well as that the leaders of the hospital (e.g., human resources director, CEO) will pursue the investigation.

3. *What are the values?* Mariana's concerns are to provide accurate information while being mindful of justice (treating employees fairly and with respect) and her responsibility to be loyal to the hospital and community (corporate citizenship).

4. *What are my options?* In the case study, Mariana could do nothing and refuse to talk with the reporter, but her job is to communicate with the media under her supervisor's counsel to ensure the accuracy and appropriateness of the information she shares.

5. *What should I do?* Mariana should tell the truth; she should talk to the media and offer accurate information regarding the case. Nonetheless, she must be careful not to discuss the coder or the physicians specifically because they have employee rights.

6. *What justified my choice?* If Mariana carries out her job as she should, her choice will be justified by adherence to and respect for the ethical principles of justice, fidelity, beneficence, and autonomy in the healthcare environment. Her actions will not be justified if she chooses to disclose information about clinic personnel without due process, ignore the television reporter's text message, or give misleading information.

7. *How can I prevent this ethical problem?* Mariana's primary role is communication. She could contribute significantly to future in-house communications designed to educate hospital employees about ethical standards and institutional integrity.

William Nelson, former chief of the Ethics Education Service in the National Center for Ethics in Health Care, offers an ethical decision-making tool based on the concept of procedural justice. Similar to Glover's, Nelson's (2005) model is a step process:

1. *Clarify the ethical conflict, first by determining whether the conflict is actually an ethical one.* A healthcare professional should be able to identify what the ethical issue is. If he/she cannot, the problem should be referred to another person. For example, if the question is "purely legal," he/she should consult with the healthcare organization's attorney (Nelson 2005, 11).

2. *Identify all affected stakeholders.* In the case study, the ethical issues raised many concerns. Medicare's investigation of fraud brings the hospital's integrity into question, and the physicians' actions incite financial issues and concerns. Furthermore, any actions taken must consider the public—community members' perception of the hospital as doing no harm and acting ethically. Mariana must be mindful of procedural justice and honesty regarding all stakeholders to ensure that communications via the media are accurate, timely, and true.

3. *Understand the circumstances surrounding the ethical conflict.* The financial arrangement between AMU and the clinic's physician leaders may be a basis of the conflict in the case study. The situation may also be cause for speculation: If Medicare finds that fraud is occurring in the SportsMed clinic, could it be occurring in other AMU clinics? Or, why did it occur in one clinic

and not the others? These questions are to be addressed by AMU's leaders. It would not be appropriate for Mariana to lead the fact-finding mission, given her job responsibilities. She is in charge of communications regarding the investigation.

4. *Identify the ethical perspectives relevant to the conflict.* Mariana is expected to uphold the standards of fidelity and justice and communicate appropriately. For the other leaders (i.e., the attorney, the CFO, and the CEO), fiduciary responsibility is pertinent as well.

5. *Identify different options for action.* Mariana could do nothing; communicate too much information; or—obviously the best choice—act ethically by communicating the facts, engaging in future actions decided by AMU's leaders, and responding to external events (Medicare's investigation) as well as internal policies (audits of the clinic's operations).

6. *Select among the options.* The following epilogue demonstrates this step: Medicare found that the clinic had indeed engaged in fraudulent practices, and the government agency took legal action. One of the three original physician owners retired from the profession, announcing that he wanted to "spend more time with family." AMU renegotiated its contract with the other two physician leaders, who agreed to forgo their profit share and receive only a salary. AMU paid Medicare the monies owed plus a penalty. Regarding AMU policy, the human resources department—in close counsel with the hospital's attorney—designed in-house training and implemented it with Mariana's assistance. Via the in-house newsletter, Mariana communicated that all employees were to participate in a four-hour workshop on ethical decision making to learn how to address ethical issues. She also communicated with the media, staying mindful of employee rights as well as the need to share accurate information. She reported that Medicare had concluded that the coding practices were inaccurate and that AMU was taking steps to ensure that this infraction was addressed appropriately. In addition, AMU planned to conduct more frequent audits of its departments and clinics without advance notice. The coder who informed Medicare of the fraud resigned from the clinic, citing that other employees were not as kind to her as they had been in the past, and accepted a job in a neighboring town at a physician practice not affiliated with AMU.

7. *Share and implement the decision.* Mariana did not communicate with the media until she received direction from AMU's leaders. She then replied to the television reporter, stating that the investigation was underway and

that she would be communicative after AMU gathered the facts. Mariana remained the "go to" person for media inquiries throughout the investigation and subsequent activities.

8. *Review the decision to ensure it achieved the desired goal.* AMU regularly trains its employees in ethical practices and conducts more frequent audits of its departments and clinics. It offered to transfer the coder to another AMU facility, but she did not accept the offer.

HEALTHCARE MARKETERS AND ETHICS ASSESSED

Persons in positions of responsibility and power may find themselves in challenging situations similar to the events at the Atlantic SportsMed clinic. ACHE offers a self-assessment tool designed to help leaders identify their ethical strengths and note areas for improvement. This exercise is reflective, not one to share or to use to rank others. The assessment questions address one's thoughts and beliefs regarding leadership and relationships with the community, patients and their families, the governing board, colleagues and staff, clinicians, buyers, payers, and suppliers. The topics and situations addressed by the self-assessment are outlined on ACHE's website.

CHAPTER QUESTIONS

1. A celebrity has been admitted to your clinic. The media have somehow heard about it and have contacted you for information. What should you do? How should you respond? What should you not do? Why/why not?
2. In the table of ethical/legal behavior below, in which quadrant would you place the behavior of the coder who reported the discrepancies to the Medicare Fraud Control Units? Why did you select the cell you did?

Action	Unethical	Ethical
Illegal		
Legal		

3. Review the codes of ethics of two healthcare professions (e.g., such the codes posted on ACHE's and AHIMA's websites). What do they have in common? In what ways are they different?

CHAPTER EXERCISES

1. *Ethical decision making*

   You are the marketing officer at Sullivan's Island Medical University. Three employees work in your department—you, the marketing director (your boss, who oversees all marketing/public relations duties), and the marketing media officer (your colleague, who oversees all communications to external audiences). You oversee all in-house communications (i.e., for audiences inside the medical school). Currently, you are writing articles about new residents who have just arrived at Sullivan's Island Medical University for their surgical rotations. Your articles will be published in the in-house newsletter *Take Note* in a recurring section titled "Welcome to Our New Docs." The articles about the new residents include their educational background and some personal information, such as marital status, the names and ages of their children, and their hobbies. To prepare for your interview with resident Patricia Gray, you google her name and find her Facebook page. The photos, captions, and comments on her page indicate that she is a big partier; in several of the photos, she obviously is drinking alcohol. One photo shows her pouring champagne on the head of another woman. Another shows her holding a beer can in one hand and giving the thumbs-up signal with the other. Moreover, she uses profanity throughout her posts.

   a. In your position as a marketer in a hospital, do you think Dr. Gray's Facebook page is an issue that warrants your attention? Why or why not?

   b. With reference to the four quadrants model presented in Exhibit 4.1, define where you think this scenario should be classified.

   c. Using one of the ethical decision-making models explained in the chapter, explain how you would address this situation.

   d. How do you think the AMA policy about physicians and the use of social media (summarized at the top of page 52) relates to Dr. Gray's Facebook page?

The AMA (2010) social media policy encourages physicians to

Use privacy settings to safeguard personal information and content to the fullest extent possible on social networking sites.

Routinely monitor their own Internet presence to ensure that the personal and professional information on their own sites and content posted about them by others [are] accurate and appropriate.

Maintain appropriate boundaries of the patient–physician relationship when interacting with patients online and ensure patient privacy and confidentiality is maintained.

Consider separating personal and professional content online.

Recognize that actions online and content posted can negatively affect their reputations among patients and colleagues and may even have consequences for their medical careers.

2. *Health Insurance Portability and Accountability Act (HIPAA) and George Clooney's medical records*

On September 21, 2007, actor George Clooney was treated at Palisades Medical Center in New Jersey for injuries incurred from a motorcycle accident. Twenty-seven employees—none of whom was a care provider for Clooney—logged into the hospital's electronic health record (EHR) system and viewed Clooney's medical records. Their actions were discovered after a routine audit. All 27 employees were suspended for four weeks without pay (Goldman 2007).

a. Explain why the 27 employees' actions were HIPAA violations.

b. With reference to the four quadrants model presented in Exhibit 4.1, define where you think this scenario should be classified.

c. Explain why a HIPAA violation is an ethical issue.

d. Why does Palisades Medical Center conduct audits of EHR use?

e. Suppose you are Palisades Medical Center's public relations/marketing officer.

➤ What do you say to the news media when they ask for the names of the 27 employees?

➤ What information would you include in a press release to be read by the public as well as by the employees of Palisades Medical Center?

A Note Regarding HIPAA and Palisades Medical Center

Congress passed HIPAA in 1996 to address patients' right to confidentiality in healthcare settings. Of relevance to this case is the rule that protects patients' privacy and requires providers to ensure confidentiality and identify and protect against "reasonably anticipated" disclosures of personal information (see www .hhs.gov/ocr/privacy).

REFERENCES

American Medical Association (AMA). 2010. "New AMA Policy Helps Guide Physicians' Use of Social Media." News release, November 8. www.ama-assn.org/ama/pub/news/news /social-media-policy.page.

Beauchamp, T. L., and J. F. Childress. 2001. *Principles of Biomedical Ethics*, fifth edition. New York: Oxford University Press.

Cellucci, L., and C. Wiggins. 2010. *Essential Techniques for Healthcare Managers*. Chicago: Health Administration Press.

Dessler, G. 2009. *Fundamentals of Human Resource Management: Content, Competencies, and Applications*. Upper Saddle River, NJ: Prentice Hall.

Glover, J. 2006. "Ethical Decision-Making Guidelines and Tools." In *Ethical Challenges in the Management of Health Information*, second edition, edited by L. Harman, 33–50. Sudbury, MA: Jones and Bartlett.

Goldberg, H. S. 1963. *Hippocrates, Father of Medicine*. New York: Franklin Watts.

Goldman, R. 2007. "Clooney Proves Private Health Records Not So Private." *ABC News* October 11. http://abcnews.go.com/US/story?id=3714207&page=2.

Henderson, V. E. 1982. "The Ethical Side of Enterprise." *Sloan Management Review (Pre-1986)* 23 (3): 37–47.

National Commission for the Protection of Human Subjects of Biomedical and Behavioral Research. 1979. *The Belmont Report: Ethical Principles and Guidelines for the Protection of Human Subjects of Research*. www.shrm.org/templatestools/hrqa/pages/cananemployer rescindajoboffer.aspx.

Nelson, W. 2005. "An Organizational Ethics Decision-Making Process." *Healthcare Executive* 20 (4): 9–14.

Rawls, J. 1971. *A Theory of Justice*. Cambridge, MA: Belknap Press.

Winkler, E., and R. Gruen. 2005. "First Principles: Substantive Ethics for Healthcare Organizations." *Journal of Healthcare Management* 50 (2): 109–19.

THE FIVE Ps OF HEALTHCARE MARKETING

FEATURE CASE: MARKET MANAGEMENT

This real-life case invites students to analyze and prioritize various kinds of information common to a dynamic and competitive healthcare marketplace as part of an organization's strategic marketing process. It presents the unique and important issues and challenges a regional healthcare provider (Community Medical Centers) had to face as it attempted to engage patients, physicians, payers, and the general public in a politically sensitive environment. This case reinforces the material introduced in Part II of this text by asking students to assume the role of assistant director of strategic planning and marketing and to analyze, synthesize, and prioritize findings from Community Medical Centers' recent environmental assessment to position the organization and promote its services to area physicians, patients, payers, and the general public.

Information included in this case was derived from the *California Health Care Almanac*, a publication of the California HealthCare Foundation (2009). Although the information about the Fresno, California, healthcare market is true to fact, modifications have been made to names, roles, settings, and numerical values to preserve anonymity and accentuate points of learning.

INTRODUCTION

Twenty-three-year-old Rachel McKee completed her undergraduate degree in healthcare administration with an emphasis in planning and marketing. To her delight, she was offered the position of assistant director of strategic planning and marketing at Community Medical Centers (CMC), a large healthcare organization in central California. Rachel was ambitious and eager to make an early impact. She was pleased that her new boss and mentor, Lindsey Chadwick—a seasoned healthcare veteran—seemed confident in Rachel's ability to process complex information and assume increasingly important responsibilities.

Lindsey understood the intricacies of CMC and the local healthcare market. Her supervisor and members of the board had put her in charge of updating the organization's strategic marketing plan in response to important, ongoing changes in the local and regional markets. Lindsey assigned Rachel the important task of performing an environmental assessment and using the results to complete a strengths, weaknesses, opportunities, and threats (SWOT) analysis and draft a summary of the organization's core strategic initiatives. From these important documents, Lindsey and Rachel would update CMC's strategic marketing plan.

From the outset, Lindsey advised Rachel to gather and assess relevant market information from various sources, including noted health industry publications; organization, statewide, and other publicly available databases; and interviews with executives, physician groups, insurance companies, regulators, and others. Like an investigative reporter, Rachel was directed to probe and dig for important and useful information that would ultimately provide a framework and justification for the organization's marketing plan. From her coursework in college, Rachel remembered that a marketing plan must include timely and accurate information about a market's healthcare providers—notably hospitals and local physicians. She knew that a summary of key market demographics, including patient, employer, and insurance company profiles, was essential. A broad yet detailed understanding of the public at large and the political dynamics among the provider community also was vital. Finally, she needed to gain an overview of key industry trends. After four months of diligent study, networking, and thoughtful analysis, Rachel presented her environmental assessment to Lindsey. Her assessment included the following highlights.

FRESNO MARKET BACKGROUND

With a total population of 1.6 million people, the greater Fresno area had seen strong growth over the past decade—up 22 percent compared to 14 percent statewide. It was one of the poorest communities in California; the incomes of nearly half of the Fresno area population were below 200 percent of the federal poverty level. Educational attainment was also well below the state average; only 22 percent of adults held a college degree. Approximately 50 percent of the market population were Latino, 37.5 percent were white (non-Latino), and 20 percent were foreign born. The health status of local/regional residents was generally not good; approximately 20 percent self-reported fair or poor health status, and more than 27 percent were living with asthma, diabetes, or both. The unemployment rate in the area was high and continuing to rise; 15.5 percent of the population was out of work (up 5 percent over the previous year and 5 percent higher than the statewide average). Although agriculture was a vital part of the local and regional economies, the largest employers in the market were public-sector organizations, including Fresno County, the City of Fresno, and the Fresno school district. Two major healthcare systems—CMC and Saint Agnes Medical Center—were among the area's largest private employers (California HealthCare Foundation 2009).

HOSPITAL/HEALTH SYSTEM PROVIDERS

Most of the hospitals in the region were not-for-profit or government/district hospitals. The Fresno community had an acute care bed capacity of 173 per 100,000 (slightly less than the statewide average of 182) and an occupancy rate of 68 percent (greater than the statewide average of 59 percent). The major hospitals ran near capacity at certain times of the year.

The major hospital systems in Fresno County were CMC (800 beds across three hospitals), Saint Agnes Medical Center (more than 400 beds), and Kaiser Permanente Fresno Medical Center (165 beds). These hospital systems represented roughly 50, 30, and 10 percent of the hospital market, respectively. CMC and Saint Agnes served a large geographic area and enjoyed a referral base from several outlying counties. Historically, the relationship between CMC and Saint Agnes had been characterized by little collaboration and intense, long-standing competition bordering on animosity. While Saint Agnes was located in the more affluent part of north Fresno and was often described as the "cash cow" of its 40-hospital parent corporation, CMC's 500-bed flagship facility was located in the heart of Fresno and, with its nine outpatient clinics, served as Fresno County's primary safety net provider.[1] Financial losses at CMC's flagship facility were largely offset by highly profitable operations at its two sister hospitals located in more affluent communities to the north and northeast. In recent years, CMC had reversed its negative financial performance and had become modestly profitable.

Reports from the Office of Statewide Health Planning and Development indicated an increasingly unfavorable payer mix across all Fresno area hospitals—an indication of the community's high levels of poverty, lack of insurance, and Medi-Cal (similar to Medicaid) coverage. The Saint Agnes payer base was approximately 25 percent Medi-Cal. CMC—with its more than 30-year contract with Fresno County to provide indigent care—reported that nearly 40 percent of its patients were covered by Medi-Cal. Major initiatives at CMC included the recent opening of 160 new beds at its flagship hospital, including 56 neonatal intensive care beds. After opening a new patient tower, Saint Agnes added 36 neurosurgery and critical care beds. In some cases, new hospital construction was a response to both capacity issues and compliance with state seismic standards. Both CMC and Saint Agnes also added new programs to stem the exodus of patients to out-of-area providers of services not previously offered within the community.

Survey respondents' characterizations of the quality of care at Fresno area hospitals ranged from poor to good. Many opted to leave the area when they got "really sick"; a study showed that patients sought nearly $500 million in medical care services outside the greater Fresno area annually for a variety of reasons, notably long wait times, physician shortages, and concerns about the quality of care provided by area hospitals. In recent years, area hospitals aligned themselves with academic teaching programs to support clinical/medical training programs, improve the quality of care, enhance their reputations, and recruit more physicians to the market. Notable associations included CMC's formal affiliation with the University of California, San Francisco, and Saint Agnes's affiliation with Stanford University for cardiology and neurosciences.

Although Saint Agnes was widely regarded as the premier hospital in the market, highly publicized recent outbreaks of methicillin-resistant staphylococcus aureus (MRSA) infections and Legionnaires' disease had raised questions about its patient care and quality.

PHYSICIAN AND ALLIED HEALTH COMMUNITY

The greater Fresno area suffered from a notable shortage of primary care and specialist physicians, with 45 primary care physicians per 100,000 residents versus 59 statewide and 118 physicians overall per 100,000 residents versus 174 statewide. An aging physician workforce led market observers to expect shortages to worsen. Nurses and other allied health personnel were also in short supply, causing the federal government to classify most of the market as a health professional shortage area. Primary and specialty physician shortages invariably resulted in long appointment wait times—a key reason many insured patients sought medical care outside the local market. Wait times for dermatologic appointments, for example, were reportedly 9 to 12 months. Other specialists in short supply included neurosurgeons, general surgeons, cardiologists, gastroenterologists, oncologists, otolaryngologists, ophthalmologists, and psychiatrists.

Recruiting new physicians to the Fresno area was challenging because of various factors, including poor payer mix, poor reimbursement, ongoing hospital call coverage obligations, and quality-of-life considerations. Although many physicians already established in the market were overworked, they were apprehensive about losing market share and thus had little interest in recruiting. Many respondents reported that the physician shortage would have been even more acute if it were not for the many foreign-born physicians practicing in the Fresno area, notably natives of India and Pakistan. Many of these physicians were attracted by the area's sizable ethnic communities and focused their practices on patients from their own ethnic background.

For various reasons, Fresno had few large physician practices. Most physicians opted to practice solo or in small groups of fewer than five physicians, and single-specialty rather than multispecialty groups were the dominant practice type. Although many community physicians maintained admitting and practice privileges at multiple hospitals, they generally concentrated their practice at one hospital. For years, emergency call coverage had been a source of friction between area hospitals and physicians due to the expensive stipends hospitals had to pay to get physicians to provide call coverage.

Unlike in many markets in California and elsewhere, formal integration between physicians and hospitals was limited. Relationships generally were marked by strain and distrust. In recent years, CMC's relationships with its primary physician groups had improved, whereas Saint Agnes's hospital–physician relationships had deteriorated. Hospitals' efforts to attract and align area physicians were focused on joint ventures, many of which failed.

Area physicians' lack of loyalty to area hospitals was evidenced by the extensive movement of various services—including imaging, orthopedics, plastic surgery, and endoscopy—out of hospitals and into physician offices or physician-owned facilities. Many reports suggested that physicians' ongoing dissatisfaction with area hospitals was the basis of this activity.

PAYER/INSURANCE COMMUNITY

In contrast to other California markets, the greater Fresno area only modestly embraced managed care. Even at their peak in the mid-1990s, health maintenance organizations (HMOs) and their variants never achieved dominance in the Fresno area, and their presence shrank from roughly 30 percent in 2000 to 25 percent today. According to one report, the absence of a strong HMO/managed care presence meant that health system features common to other communities—formation of large multispecialty physician groups, close hospital–physician alignment, provider familiarity with performance measurement and reporting, and aggressive care and utilization management—were not pervasive in the Fresno market.

Only 46 percent of area residents (compared to 59 percent statewide) had private medical insurance, and 16 percent were uninsured. Medi-Cal enrollment was high in the Fresno area, at approximately 30 percent. Fresno's safety net was generally considered weak, fragmented, and inadequate for the needs of the population. Indeed, healthcare was considered a low priority for many of the area's county governments. Blue Shield of California and Anthem Blue Cross were the leading health insurers in the greater Fresno market. As in other regional markets, these health plans were under high pressure to moderate premiums. Many believed that doing so would be extremely challenging in the face of escalating hospital costs. Because some hospitals—notably Saint Agnes and CMC's Clovis Community Medical Center—were considered "must haves" by employer purchasers, these hospitals had strong negotiating leverage with area health plans.

THE FUTURE OF HEALTHCARE: KEY INDUSTRY TRENDS

Rachel recognized that healthcare is a dynamic and ever-changing industry whose future is difficult to predict. Her assessment summarized the key trends that would likely define healthcare's immediate future.

THE ECONOMY

Although the economy was slowly improving, it was expected to remain fragile due to continued high unemployment in the United States and Europe. The national economy was expected to impact both demand and supply dimensions of the healthcare industry (Valentine and Masters 2012).

HEALTHCARE REFORM

Various elements of the Affordable Care Act were implemented on schedule, including ventures into bundled payment, accountable care organizations (ACOs), and value-based purchasing activities. State health insurance exchanges loomed around the corner; many were in active development. This trend—with its focus on benefits and network development—needed to be monitored (Valentine and Masters 2012).

HOSPITAL–PHYSICIAN ALIGNMENT

Physician employment was expected to remain the preferred approach to hospital–physician alignment. Some physician/medical groups would still favor independence, and most hospitals/health systems would need to balance a dual approach to meeting the needs of both independent and employed physicians. The need to clinically integrate employed and independent physicians would remain critical if hospitals/health systems expected to respond effectively to healthcare reform (Valentine and Masters 2012).

REVENUES AND EXPENSES

Per unit revenues (e.g., average net revenue per procedure or per patient day) were expected to increase at a rate slower than cost trends over the next 12 to 24 months. Medicare payments would increase by less than 2 percent, and most states were expected to hold the line on Medicaid payments (or even reduce reimbursement rates). Commercial payers would likely limit rate increases to 4 to 6 percent. Some payers, including Medicare, were expected to tie certain rate increases to documented quality improvements. Value-based purchasing, bundled payments, readmission rate reductions, ACOs, and other risk-based arrangements would present opportunities for greater financial reward for low-cost, high-quality providers. Reducing costs would remain a top priority in the coming fiscal years. Simultaneously, it was expected that patient throughput and occupancy levels would need to increase in both acute care/hospital-based and outpatient settings to maximize economies of scale (i.e., reduction of per unit cost resulting from high volume) and use of resources (Valentine and Masters 2012).

ACCESS TO CAPITAL

Access to capital (funds) would continue to be a key catalyst for mergers, sales, affiliations, and other alliances among hospitals. Capital was expected to be more difficult to obtain in the immediate future due to the weak economy, lower patient volumes, and deteriorating payer mix. Most independent hospital boards would continue to ask whether they could remain independent and, if so, whether they should (Valentine and Masters 2012).

INFORMATION TECHNOLOGY

Useful data that could inform clinical and financial decisions in real time would become key to increasing revenues and managing expenses more effectively. Information technology systems and strategies would need to be sufficiently robust to capture large volumes of data that could be readily integrated into decision making (clinical and financial) and marketing efforts (Valentine and Masters 2012).

CONSOLIDATIONS, CLOSURES, ALLIANCES, AND MERGERS

The healthcare reform agenda was expected to continue, with 5 percent of acute care hospitals closing by 2020. Further consolidation and alignment of hospitals and medical groups was expected as these entities joined together to improve access to capital, form ACOs, and achieve cost reductions through economies of scale (Valentine and Masters 2012).

CLINICAL INTEGRATION AND CARE DELIVERY REDESIGN

Processes associated with clinical integration and care delivery redesign were within the "golden triangle" of cost containment, quality improvement, and financial performance. Future success factors for clinical integration and care delivery redesign included attention to all points of the care continuum: coordination of primary care, acute care, and post–acute care (Valentine and Masters 2012).

WORKFORCE ISSUES

Pressure to reduce operating costs from 10 to 20 percent over the next three to five years was expected to continue. The enormity of this reduction would mandate further reducing nonclinical staffing, outsourcing functions to less costly vendors, and reducing wages or holding wages flat and adjusting benefit plans. Backlash from organized labor (i.e., unions) was expected (Valentine and Masters 2012).

Smart Growth

Inpatient and selective outpatient use rates were expected to decline in the immediate/intermediate future because of continued high unemployment, shifting the costs of health-related benefits from employers to employees, increased price shopping among patients seeking to obtain health services at the lowest cost, and postponing nonessential medical care. Accordingly, healthcare leadership teams would need to identify ways to selectively grow their organizations' market share in areas that would improve their profitability (Valentine and Masters 2012).

Next Steps

Lindsey was pleased with the substance and quality of Rachel's environmental assessment. The task of analyzing, synthesizing, and prioritizing these findings—including developing a summary of strategic issues and marketing plans—lay ahead.

Note

1. The term *safety net provider* generally refers to providers (including hospitals and physicians) who offer government-financed programs that enable people to receive healthcare services when they cannot pay for them due to a lack of private resources. For example, Medicaid becomes a safety net for long-term care services after a patient has exhausted his/her private funds.

Discussion Questions

1. According to Rachel's environmental assessment, what were CMC's most important strengths, weaknesses, opportunities, and threats?
2. Identify and describe CMC's most important strategic issues.
3. In what ways should CMC's strategic issues have driven the development of a strategic marketing plan?

4. What are the foremost issues Rachel and Lindsey should have considered as they positioned CMC and promoted its services to area physicians, patients, payers, and the general public?
5. After completing the environmental assessment—including the SWOT analysis and summary of strategic issues—Lindsey and Rachel needed to develop business and marketing plans to advance the organization's strategic initiatives. In your judgment, what are the elements or characteristics of a valid marketing plan?

REFERENCES

California HealthCare Foundation. 2009. "Fresno: Poor Economy, Poor Health Stress an Already Fragmented System." *California Health Care Almanac* regional markets issue brief, July. www.chcf.org/~/media/MEDIA%20LIBRARY%20Files/PDF/A/PDF%20AlmanacRegMktBriefFresno09.pdf.

Valentine, S. T., and G. M. Masters. 2012. "For Board Members Only: 10 Trends That Will Define Healthcare in 2012." Governance Institute E-Briefings 9 (1). Published in January. www.governanceinstitute.com/ResearchPublications/ResourceLibrary/tabid/185/CategoryID/63/List/1/Level/a/ProductID/1219/Default.aspx?SortField=DateCreated+DESC%2cDateCreated+DESC.

PHYSICIANS

After studying this chapter, you will be able to

➤ discuss medicine as a profession,

➤ explain the complex relationship between physicians and hospitals,

➤ describe converging trends that have brought about the large, complex practice arrangements among today's physicians, and

➤ identify the unique business and marketing concerns of physician group practices.

CASE STUDY: PHYSICIANS' IMAGING CENTER

Carl Shaw had been the administrator of Physicians' Imaging Center in a large and competitive metro area for three years. The Center was owned by six radiologists, who also constituted its governing board. Also located in the metro area were five larger freestanding imaging centers and three hospitals (at which all six of the Center's physicians had privileges). All provided similar services, and the market was extremely competitive. The Center had been successful and had been earning thin but consistent profits. The Center's physicians were considering the purchase of an expensive new scanner, believing it would make them more competitive.

Carl had run the numbers and determined that if the new scanner was used at maximum capacity, it would pay for itself in about three years. However, he didn't believe that the Center would be able to achieve the necessary patient volume. In addition, his reading of the literature suggested that the added medical benefit of the new technology was negligible at best. He believed that the Center would gain a greater competitive edge by using the money for projects that directly impacted patients, such as remodeling the waiting room and updating the electronic scheduling system. Nevertheless, his physicians were adamant that they needed this scanner to remain competitive.

Babett Simmons was the CEO of St. Lucy's, one of the three hospitals in the same large metro area. Five years previously, the three hospitals had been the only facilities offering imaging services in the area. Now St. Lucy's competed not only with the other two hospitals but also with the six physician-owned, freestanding imaging centers. The physician owners of the six facilities all had staff privileges at St. Lucy's. Dr. Winkel, the head of St. Lucy's radiology department, was a member of St. Lucy's board of directors and was not affiliated with any of the freestanding imaging centers. However, she had an open invitation to join three of the centers, and she just had lunch with Carl from Physicians' Imaging Center.

Dr. Winkel was avidly interested in having St. Lucy's purchase the same new expensive scanning technology that Physicians' Imaging Center was considering and had been planning to approach St. Lucy's board with the request. But after her lunch with Carl, she was having second thoughts. St. Lucy's CEO, Babett, had been hesitant to purchase the new technology because there were so many other far more pressing demands on the hospital's resources, many of which had a direct impact on the quality of care at St. Lucy's.

Radiology was one of St Lucy's most profitable services, due in large part to Dr. Winkel's excellent reputation, vision, and clinical/management expertise. St. Lucy's could not afford to lose Dr. Winkel. The hospital's active rumor mill had just informed Babett that Physicians' Imaging Center was wooing Dr. Winkel and would soon likely steal her.

PHYSICIANS

Physicians are the most powerful clinical professionals in healthcare. They are not the largest group of healthcare professionals, but they have the broadest **licensure**. Licensure of health professionals differs from state to state, but in most states physicians are allowed to administer all healthcare treatments and modalities, other than fill prescriptions. Physicians directly and indirectly oversee all health professionals and their work. In many states, for example, physical therapists cannot treat patients without a physician's order, just as imaging professionals cannot take X-rays unless directed to do so by a physician and just as pharmacists cannot provide medication without a physician's prescription. Nearly any duty that a nurse or therapist performs can legally be performed by a physician. That is not to say that physicians actually perform all the duties and tasks of other health professionals; indeed, most physicians are well aware of their educational and skill limits and would not attempt to provide care outside their area of expertise.

Traditionally, **medicine** has been considered one of the three fundamental professions (the other two being academics and law). According to Merriam-Webster's online dictionary, a **profession** is a principal calling or vocation based on specialized knowledge that is usually attained through long, intensive academic study. It is far more than just a job. A profession defines the education required of its members, is self-monitoring, and has its own set of ethical standards. The concept of professions has a great bearing on the field of medicine. From the television personalities of Dr. Welby in the 1960s to Dr. House in the 2000s, most people have a preconceived notion of what a physician is, what a physician does, and how a physician should act. Few people, however, have a true understanding of the changes that have occurred in the profession of medicine in the past generation alone.

BECOMING A PHYSICIAN

Medicine has always been one of the most highly respected professions. Physicians are universally regarded as smart, capable, duty bound, and—until recently—some of the most affluent in society. For the most part, people know the difficulties of applying to, being accepted into, and surviving medical school; it is a prized rite of passage. Because healthcare and healing are so valued and vital to society, medical school is highly subsidized by the state and federal governments. What many people don't know is that becoming a physician is not only an educational process; it is also a "**culturization**" process. The seminal work *Boys in White: Student Culture in Medical School* (Becker et al. 1961) describes how "boys in white"—medical students—become doctors. They enter medical school, a world of its own in which it is vitally important to determine and meet professors' expectations; study and work though intense, competitive schedules; and—through peer pressure and example—assimilate medical values. While many of the particulars of the book are dated—no longer are medical students only boys in white—its concepts remain pertinent today.

---

licensure
state laws or codes that delineate the scope of practice of specific professions and give qualified professionals who pass a proficiency exam the legal right to practice their trade

medicine
the profession of healing and caregiving as provided by licensed physicians

profession
a principal calling or vocation based on specialized knowledge that is usually attained through long, intensive academic study

"culturization"
learning and adopting the activity and behavior deemed appropriate or required of a specific group or profession

Just like 50 years ago, women and men enter medical school as bright, aspiring students and emerge four years later as doctors. Over those four years, they are taught a way of thinking, a way of diagnosing diseases and conditions, and a way of treating patients. However, those strenuous four years—called (rather confusingly) **undergraduate medical education**—are just the beginning. While medical school graduates have earned the title of physician, in today's complex medical world they also need to complete multiyear specialization training—internships and residencies—called **graduate medical education (GME)**. No longer does someone fresh out of medical school expect to go directly into practice. The length of GME depends on the specialty. At one end of the spectrum is family medicine, which usually requires three years of GME; at the other end is neurosurgery, which requires completion of a one-year internship and a residency program of at least five years. Physicians wishing to subspecialize need to complete even more years of training in their chosen discipline, and even then, completion of a GME residency may not be the end. Residency graduates can choose to sit for arduous **board certification** exams in their chosen specialty. After passing the exam and becoming board certified, they must complete and document continuing medical education yearly or lose their certification.

Physicians and Hospitals

While much of what physicians do occurs in their offices, they need to have access to hospitals to treat seriously ill patients and perform procedures that cannot be done in the office (due to equipment, personnel, and even zoning laws). To practice at a hospital, a physician needs to apply for **medical staff privileges**. The majority of physicians do not apply for jobs at hospitals or become hospital employees; they ask to become privileged members of hospital medical staffs. Because hospitals are responsible and at risk for any and all procedures and treatments performed in their facilities, it behooves them to closely scrutinize any physician asking for privileges. This process, called **credentialing**, involves collecting and evaluating a physician applicant's education records, work history, malpractice history, legal history, and letters of reference and running a criminal background check. Many hospitals have a team of employees specifically for this purpose. If the team finds that all is in order, the hospital's medical chief of staff recommends to the hospital's board of directors that the physician be granted medical staff privileges.

A strange relationship exists between physicians and hospitals. For the most part, physicians are not employees of a hospital and so are not under the supervision or direction of the hospital's administrative personnel; the administrators and managers have no direct power over the physicians practicing at their hospital or over their work. (As mentioned earlier in the chapter, true professions are self-monitoring.) Physicians on staff report to the hospital's medical chief of staff, who also is not a hospital employee. If the hospital's administrators (or its board of directors) want to remove a physician's privileges, they must ask the medical chief of staff to do so.

---

undergraduate medical education
medical school, usually four years in duration

graduate medical education (GME)
the years of internships, residencies, and additional training and specialization following graduation from medical school

board certification
an official status reflecting mastery of a specialty, granted by professional agencies and organizations to physicians who pass an advanced examination; maintained by yearly completion and documentation of continuing medical education

medical staff privileges
permission to practice in a hospital, granted to physicians who pass the hospital's credentialing process

All other caregivers are usually hospital employees and work under the direction of the physicians, who are not hospital employees; no care or treatments can be provided in a hospital without a physician's orders or approval. Thus, hospitals are utterly dependent on physicians to admit and care for patients; without patient revenues, hospitals cannot exist. Hospitals cannot do business—cannot provide any care at all—without physicians.

This mutual dependence engenders a peculiar and rather uneven power dynamic. Physicians need a place to practice, and they often hold privileges in many or all of the hospitals in an area. As hospital executives are well aware, physicians who are not pleased with one hospital can simply admit their patients to a different hospital, which will be more than happy to accept the additional business and meet that physician's wants, needs, and—sometimes—demands. Hospital executives and the boards they report to walk a tight and sometimes precarious line between fulfilling their legal obligations of fiscal responsibility, ensuring that all care delivered in the facility is appropriate and of excellent quality, and keeping the physicians happy. Ensuring that physicians engage with the hospital closely enough to admit their patients to it exclusively is called **physician bonding**. Hospitals devote a large proportion of their resources and efforts to making their facilities convenient and pleasant for physicians. For example, most hospitals provide physicians with their own lounges, lunch rooms, parking places, telephones, computers, and lab coats. Hospitals regularly subsidize physician office buildings (which are often located nearby) to relieve physicians of the pressures of finding and maintaining their own practice sites and give them easy access to hospital equipment, technology, and personnel. Unhappy physicians who have established their practices in a hospital's office building have greater difficulty moving their business and patients elsewhere than do unhappy physicians set up in non-hospital-subsidized offices.

In all businesses, some products are more profitable than others, and so is the case with hospitals and medical care. Hospitals work hard to live up to their missions and to provide excellent care to all patients, but a hospital would be foolish not to bond most closely with physicians who provide the most profitable services. Thus, physicians who do highly technical work, are in shortage, or are generously reimbursed have particular power in hospitals. These physicians' wants, needs, and demands often receive the most attention and are most often met.

This discussion brings up a question that is posed often in this text and perhaps the most important question in healthcare marketing: Who is the customer? Patients, whom one would intuitively think of as a hospital's customers, cannot receive care in a hospital without being admitted by a physician. Because hospitals are completely dependent on physicians, they often treat physicians more like customers than they do patients. Physicians are hospital customers whose wants and needs must be met or they will take their business and their patients elsewhere. But physicians are not customers in the true sense; they do not purchase goods or services from hospitals. They work at hospitals essentially for free while hospitals provide them with staff, equipment, and space. Still, as long

credentialing
an in-depth background, education, and practice investigation performed by a hospital to determine whether a physician is qualified to receive medical staff privileges

physician bonding
ensuring that physicians engage with a hospital closely enough to admit their patients to it exclusively

as hospitals need physicians to admit their patients, this peculiar quasi-customer power dynamic will continue to characterize hospital–physician relations.

PHYSICIANS AND PHYSICIAN PRACTICES

In the past, most physicians worked in solo practice or in small groups of two to three physicians. While some specializations lent themselves to larger groups, physician groups of more than five physicians were rare. The convention is not so today. A number of converging trends have contributed to the formation of larger, more complex practice arrangements among physicians. These trends include but are not limited to hospitals' involvement in group practices, the advent of managed care, the increasing complexity of medicine, and decreasing reimbursement from both public and private insurers.

Running a practice is essentially running a business, and medical schools traditionally have done little to prepare physicians for the world of business. Maintaining a medical office facility is expensive and far more complex than most people realize. For example, in addition to practicing medicine, physician owners need to

- ♦ meet zoning laws and public health regulations;

- ♦ adhere to laws and regulations regarding the hiring and employment of a variety of personnel, including nurses and receptionists;

- ♦ establish payroll, accounting, and tax procedures;

- ♦ ensure an adequate inventory of medicines, medical equipment, treatments, and materials;

- ♦ ensure sterilization and septic conditions throughout the facility;

- ♦ create a welcoming office and waiting area;

- ♦ tend to building needs and upkeep; and

- ♦ engage in timely insurance reimbursement processes.

One form of physician bonding in particular—hospitals' subsidization of physician offices—is an attractive alternative for physicians in practice; it leaves many of a practice's business chores and duties to hospital personnel and enables physicians to focus on practicing medicine. Some hospitals also supply nurses and office managers, administrative personnel, accountants, and even computer systems. As hospitals became increasingly involved with physician groups in the 1980s and 1990s, they became interested in integrating with them. Some large hospitals bought physician group practices, which made the physicians hospital employees. The purchase of physician practices resolved a number of political issues for hospitals, but the popularity of this arrangement was short lived, and it did not become the dominant model of physician practice.

At the same time hospitals became interested in physician practices, **health maintenance organizations (HMOs)** and **managed care** were emerging as a new model for healthcare delivery. This model required physicians to contract with HMOs or managed care organizations to provide care to a specific group of patients for a predetermined monthly reimbursement. Because physicians received only a specific, predetermined monthly amount per enrolled patient regardless of the care or services provided to each patient, this contractual arrangement put physicians at financial risk. Physicians found that they had strengthened negotiating power over their reimbursement levels when they joined together and formed large bargaining groups called **independent practice associations (IPAs)**. For physicians, a side benefit of IPAs was access to a close, built-in network of peers with whom they could consult regarding patient and practice issues. At the same time, the male-dominated medical profession was evolving into one shared by women and men. IPAs were more female and family friendly because they were able to attain economies of scale and divide duties, such as call coverage on weekends, among a large number of physicians, thereby reducing physicians' off-hour obligations and increasing their free time.

One of the current trends among physician group practices is the creation of ambulatory care centers (see Chapter 1). Physician-owned walk-in clinics, one-day surgery centers, in-office medical laboratories, sports medicine clinics, and freestanding imaging centers—to name a few—have proliferated. Traditionally these types of services were offered only by hospitals and were an important source of hospital revenue. As both public and private insurers look for ways to reduce reimbursement to both hospitals and physicians, ownership of these highly profitable services has become increasingly desirable and the ambulatory care market has become increasingly competitive. Small clinics and freestanding facilities have less overhead than hospitals do and often can provide these services at lower costs. Patients like receiving care in smaller, often homey and comfortable settings rather than in large, sterile hospitals. Physicians see this exciting opportunity as a new revenue stream in an increasingly competitive and decreasing reimbursement environment. Hospitals see it as physicians "stealing their lunch." To add insult to injury, this lunch, which has dire financial consequences for the hospital, is often eaten by the hospital's own medical staff.

Ambulatory care centers are big money and big business and almost universally need to be run by a professional team of healthcare managers. In hospitals, healthcare managers work *with* physicians, but in physician practices and physician-owned care centers, healthcare managers work *for* physicians. As in hospitals, the relationship between healthcare managers and physicians in physician-owned practices is characterized by an interesting power dynamic. Physicians have a deep understanding of the clinical care side of healthcare, and after many years of working in the healthcare industry, many believe they understand the industry's ins and outs. Healthcare managers, on the other hand, often

---

health maintenance organization (HMO)
a managed care delivery system that merges the provision of care and the reimbursement function of health insurance

managed care
a prospective reimbursement system designed to control the cost and delivery of healthcare while improving the quality and outcomes of care

independent practice association (IPA)
a loose network of physician groups and practices, often formed to increase physicians' negotiating power over HMOs and managed care organizations

have little to no understanding of clinical care but have a broad, deep, educated understanding of healthcare business. Their knowledge can sometimes conflict with physicians' narrower understanding of healthcare, which is often primarily based on their own experiences with patients and payers, not on a comprehensive understanding of the industry or on solid business skills and techniques. However, the managers are the physicians' employees and thus must find a way to reconcile these differences and work toward creating and running a profitable organization.

HEALTHCARE IS POLITICAL

Whether practicing in hospitals or physician groups, physicians want and need to take an active role in health organizations' direction and strategy. Hospitals would be foolish not to include such an influential, knowledgeable, and powerful group in its decision process. Thus, physicians are members of hospital governance; at the least, medical chiefs of staff are always members of hospitals' boards of directors. Physicians' direct and sole control of all the care provided in hospitals, however, presents a conflict of interest because they serve as voting members in the hospital governance process. Board members are ethically required to act and vote solely in the best interest of the hospital; when board decisions have a direct impact on physicians' incomes and practices, physician board members have a conflict of interest. Conversely, to strengthen their bonds with physicians, hospitals and hospital boards may placate physicians and yield to their demands, regardless of the merit of those demands.

politics

social relations involving authority or power; interests masquerading as a contest of principles or the conduct of public affairs for private advantage

The online dictionary die.net defines **politics** as "social relations involving authority or power." However, more people probably think of the definition that appears in *The Devil's Dictionary*: "a strife of interests masquerading as a contest of principles; the conduct of public affairs for private advantage" (Bierce 1993, 95). Regardless of the definition, healthcare is a politically charged environment. When Calvin Coolidge was asked why he was willing to leave his position as president of Yale University to run for president of the United States, he was said to have replied (ironically) that he wanted to get out of politics. Undoubtedly, many healthcare executives can relate to his wish.

Healthcare is political at the macro level in that it is one of the most heatedly debated topics in the United States. In one form or another, it has been an important plank in every presidential election since the 1930s. Healthcare is a complex, emotional topic; debate and differing ideas about what it is, what it should be, and how it should be paid for will be ongoing.

Likewise, healthcare is politically charged at the micro level—that is, within organizations and among health professions and professionals. Healthcare comprises myriad professions, each with its own scope of practice, code of ethics, professional associations and lobbyists, and approach to care. Most healthcare personnel are highly educated and closely identify with their chosen profession. Most aspire to independence in their work.

Healthcare is extremely hierarchical and rife with power issues and struggles, and physicians are a primary player in the game of healthcare politics.

CHAPTER QUESTIONS

1. What is a profession? What distinguishes a profession from a job?
2. Discuss the process, stages, and levels of physician education.
3. What makes the power structure in hospitals so complex? What are the roles of physicians and administrators in the power structure?
4. How have physician practices changed over the past 20 years? What are the primary causes of those changes?

CHAPTER EXERCISES

1. *Carl, the physicians, and the imaging machine*

   This chapter's case study presents a situation in which a hospital and a freestanding imaging center are competing for physicians, illustrating the power of physicians in healthcare.

   Carl, the administrator of Physicians' Imaging Center, is under pressure from his physician owners to purchase an expensive imaging machine, but he believes that the Center would gain a greater competitive edge by using the money for other purposes. Nevertheless, the physician owners are adamant that they need this scanner to remain competitive.

   Make a detailed list of all the considerations Carl must take into account in this situation. What do you recommend that Carl do?

2. *An excellent reputation*

   Babett is the CEO of St. Lucy's. Radiology is one of St. Lucy's most profitable services, due in great part to Dr. Winkel's excellent reputation, vision, and clinical/management expertise. Babett believes that Dr. Winkel likely will leave St. Lucy's soon to join Physicians' Imaging Center, but St. Lucy's cannot afford to lose Dr. Winkel.

What do you recommend that Babett do? Specifically, what information does Babett need to gather before she takes action? What are Dr. Winkel's obligations in this situation?

REFERENCES

Becker, H. S., B. Geer, E. C. Hughes, and A. Strauss. 1961. *Boys in White: Student Culture in Medical School*. Chicago: University of Chicago Press.

Bierce, A. 1993. *The Devil's Dictionary*. Mineola, NY: Dover Publications, Inc.

PATIENTS

After studying this chapter, you will be able to

➤ distinguish between patients and customers and between healthcare and medical care,

➤ identify the ways and reasons people shop and don't shop for healthcare and medical care, and

➤ explain the role of individually focused marketing communication.

CASE STUDY: WHERE SHOULD I GO? WHAT SHOULD I DO?

Matt Keller had just started his position with International, Inc., a large, multinational company. The International, Inc. human resources (HR) department held a benefits workshop on the second Tuesday of every month, so on his second day Matt was sent down to HR to learn about and select policies and plans for his benefits package. When he arrived, he found six other new employees waiting for the workshop to begin.

Jim Wheeler, the director of HR, led the workshop that day. He walked in with an armful of materials, brochures, and booklets for all the attendees. He began by welcoming everyone to International, Inc. and telling them that they needed to jump right in to be able to cover the large amount of information he had brought.

The first topic was health insurance. International, Inc. offered 12 different health plans from three different health insurance companies. Each insurance company offered bronze, silver, gold, and platinum plans ranging from bare-bones, high-deductible plans to zero-deductible, all-inclusive coverage. Some of the plans required that patients use only physicians from a preselected panel, while others allowed patients to choose any physician they wanted. Some required preauthorization for any care costing more than $300, whereas others had no authorization requirements. Some had generous health benefits with scanty dental coverage and almost nonexistent pharmacy benefits; others had generous vision and pharmacy benefits but no dental coverage. The monthly cost to the employee for these plans ranged from $3 per month to more than $400 per month.

Matt was not the only new employee who was overwhelmed with this information, and the attendees began to talk among themselves. Some of them had lived in the area for many years and shared strong opinions about the hospitals and physicians they would like to use, based on things they had heard and on their own experiences. Matt had seen billboards and advertising for local hospitals, coronary care units, and birthing centers, but these services didn't seem like the types of care he would need. He had no idea which hospitals, centers, or physicians provided the best care at the best prices or how to go about finding this kind of information.

When asked about how best to choose a plan, Jim offered this advice: "Consider any preexisting health conditions you have and any medications you take. Then make your decision from there."

Matt was 28 years old and thought of himself as very healthy. He was leaning toward the least expensive plans when one of the other new employees reminded him that young adults tended to have fewer illnesses but were far more likely to have accidents and sports injuries, which often required long hospitalizations and expensive treatments. Now Matt really didn't know what to do.

PATIENTS VERSUS CUSTOMERS

At one time, people who used healthcare services were never called or considered **customers**; they were **patients**. When healthcare organizations started to refer to their patients as customers, many caregivers were offended. *Merriam-Webster's Collegiate Dictionary* defines these terms as follows:

> pa·tient noun 1a: an individual awaiting or under medical care and treatment b: the recipient of any various personal services c: one that is acted upon
>
> cus·tom·er noun 1: one that purchases a commodity or service

Clearly, both definitions easily apply to people who use healthcare services. However, the word *patient* is passive, while the word *customer* is active.

This change from passive to active is one of the hallmarks of the changes the healthcare system has gone through in the past decades. Changing from patients to customers implies greater involvement by those receiving care and less expectation that patients will take a dependent role (i.e., physicians make all the decisions and take complete control of all care delivered while patients simply comply). But despite the token support given to patient involvement and joint decision making in today's healthcare environment, one can easily argue that after the initial decision to seek healthcare, patients and customers both are still acquiescent to physicians, their decisions, and their medical orders. Physicians are still the ones who decide what products and services will be available to the patient. And while physicians may offer patients a range of services or treatment options (including the right to refuse services), patients are rarely allowed to simply choose for themselves and purchase the treatments they want without consultation with, and authorization from, a physician.

WHAT IS THE PRODUCT?

Healthcare is an unusual product. What exactly is the product that healthcare organizations and providers sell? *Health* means different things to different people. It can be thought of as the absence of disease; the summation of many physical and medical measures (e.g., body temperature, blood pressure, cholesterol count, height, weight); or even well-being of mind, spirit, and body. Health surely means something very different to a teenage boy than it does to a 98-year-old woman.

So just what is this huge, widely diversified, and expensive industry selling? How can healthcare marketing professionals do their job if they don't know and understand the product being sold or who is using it and how? Regardless of its definition, health is far more dependent on the way people take care of themselves in terms of diet, exercise, and

---

customer
one who purchases a commodity or service

---

patient
an individual awaiting or under medical care and treatment

personal habits than on how often we visit a hospital or a physician or what kind of health insurance we have. True, the field of public health exists to ensure the health of populations and communities, but the proportion of healthcare monies spent on public health endeavors is only about 3 percent of all healthcare spending (Martin et al. 2012).

Few services in the US healthcare system are designed to help keep individuals healthy in the first place. Rather, services primarily focus on restoring health once some aspect of it has been lost. Thus, healthcare marketers need to understand that healthcare organizations and providers don't actually sell health; for the most part, they sell treatments and procedures that consumers and patients expect will restore health.

Health procedures and treatments are expensive; highly technical, life-saving procedures are often the most expensive items or services that individuals purchase over their lifetime. Healthcare services, or a lack thereof, can literally be the difference between a comfortable life and a life of pain or impairment. In many cases, they are the difference between life and death. Yet despite the magnitude of their importance, few people shop for healthcare procedures or services or have any real knowledge of the services they purchase. This unawareness poses an interesting challenge for healthcare marketers.

SHOPPING FOR HEALTHCARE

Compare the purchase of any healthcare treatment or procedure to the purchase of any other product. For most products, consumers shop using criteria such as cost, quality, ease/convenience of purchase, ease of use, and the product's potential to enhance their life or enjoyment. When a marketer knows who a product's consumers are and the criteria they use, the criteria can be the basis for informing the consumer about the product. The examples mentioned earlier in this paragraph certainly are not a definitive list of shopping criteria, but note that nearly every one of them is a misfit for healthcare.

cost as a proxy for quality
the use of cost as an indicator of a product's quality when true information regarding quality is absent; the belief that the more expensive a product is, the higher its quality

While everyone is concerned and vocal about the extremely high cost of healthcare, most people do not really want cheap care. In every other industry, sales, discounts, and low prices can be effective marketing and selling tools, but in healthcare they are likely just the opposite. Healthcare is a complex, hard-to-define, and hard-to-measure product. Even many physicians do not truly understand care and treatment outside their specialization. How, then, can patients/consumers be expected to understand the healthcare product they are purchasing? Generally, when people do not understand a product, they use **cost as a proxy for quality**. Even though there is no factual basis for this perception, most people believe that the more high-tech and expensive the physician, the treatment, or the medication, the better it is. It is difficult to imagine that a physician offering discount surgeries on Tuesdays, highly advertised seasonal sales, or BOGO (buy one, get one free) treatments would be successful. Promoting a provider as the least expensive alternative is unlikely to be an effective marketing communication strategy in healthcare.

Another unique aspect of shopping for healthcare is that accurate pricing or unambiguous information about a treatment or procedure is difficult to obtain in advance. The cost of any procedure depends on myriad factors: the patient's current health issue and preexisting conditions; the mix of personnel delivering the treatment; the location where the procedure is performed; the medications, equipment, and materials used; the type of organization performing the procedure; and the type and level of health insurance (or noninsurance) the patient has. If one calls a physician's office and simply asks how much a treatment or procedure costs, the caller is unlikely to receive a specific response. Indeed, due to the plethora of health insurance plans, most physicians do not know precisely what patients pay for their services.

Finally, a person who is sick or in critical need of care is unlikely to take the time to call three different physicians or hospitals to check and compare prices or to even care about price. While a lack of concern over price may be rational in life-or-death emergencies, people are similarly indifferent about price in nonemergency situations. For example, due to a lack of insurance or perhaps because emergency departments (EDs) are always open and appear to be convenient venues from which they cannot be turned away, a large number of patients regularly seek nonemergency care in EDs, the most expensive delivery setting, when that care should be provided in the far less expensive physician office or clinic setting.

Another facet of healthcare marketing that differs greatly from marketing in other industries is that while everyone wants health, the procedures and treatments offered by healthcare providers and organizations are often unpleasant, uncomfortable, and inconvenient. No one enjoys having his chest cut open and his ribs spread. Mammograms, pelvic exams, testicular exams, blood work, and teeth cleanings are unpleasant experiences. Even the less invasive and less painful procedures, such as imaging, can be embarrassing, uncomfortable, and inconvenient. Few people look forward to invasive surgery. At best, healthcare treatments and procedures are seen as a necessary evil.

It is a well-known adage in healthcare that a third of all coronary bypass surgeries are unnecessary, a third are questionable, and only a third are clearly needed. "According to the American Heart Association 427,000 coronary artery bypass graft (CABG) surgeries were performed in the United States in 2004, making it one of the most commonly performed major operations" (Kulick 2013). Therefore, more than 284,000 CABG procedures that year were either unnecessary or questionable. How can so many people be willing to accept their physician's opinion and undergo this highly invasive, wildly expensive, and incredibly painful and traumatic procedure? They do so because they have little information or understanding about the treatments they need and thus acquiesce to the knowledge and authority of the physician.

The role of the healthcare marketer in such situations is not to create demand for these procedures but rather to cultivate a preference in both the physician and the patient to have the procedures take place at the marketer's facility.

Choosing Healthcare

How does a patient actually choose a provider or facility? When purchasing a car or a major appliance, one can consult with any number of print and online sources to compare prices, quality, and product features. While a small number of sources offer healthcare quality and outcomes information, the data are difficult to interpret, usually not risk adjusted, and rarely used by patients and consumers (Toussaint 2012). It is close to impossible for healthcare consumers to comparison shop.

However, many people access websites that offer information (other than price and quality) about conditions, medications, and treatments. Reasons people use the Internet to search for health-related information include curiosity, not receiving enough information from their physician, or to prepare for a clinic or physician visit (AlGhamdi and Moussa 2012). The Internet is an important vehicle for health information and health marketing, and it is vital for health marketers to know who uses the Internet to search for health information and to fine-tune their message to these market segments. Some health systems are launching websites aimed at specific populations (e.g., bilingual sites for Latinos) and health apps for smartphone users (Boulton 2012). Researchers found that those who most frequently use the Internet as a source of health information are individuals aged 30 to 39 who have a university or higher education, are employed, and earn high incomes (AlGhamdi and Moussa 2012, 363).

Even in today's information age, many patients base their choice of provider on advice from family and friends (Toussaint 2012). However, the assumption that patients/consumers actually choose their providers and service locations is often misguided. Patients are regularly directed to specific providers and locations by their health insurance carriers. Even when an insurance company offers a variety of providers and locations, physicians usually steer their patients to colleagues or to the facility in which they most like to work.

Directing the Marketing Message

To whom should the healthcare marketer's efforts be directed? Patients cannot freely purchase procedures and treatments without consulting a physician. As just mentioned, patients are directed to specific facilities and panels of providers by their health insurers. Physicians decide what services, treatments, and medications their patients may obtain and funnel their patients to colleagues and to facilities in which they most like to work. Whether they are called customers, consumers, or patients, they effectively have little choice in the matter.

However, marketing messages and information fine-tuned to individuals or groups have an important place in healthcare. For example, consumers who most often choose and purchase health insurance individually (not from their employers or from the government) are the elderly, who receive **Medicare** and purchase **Medigap insurance** policies

---

Medicare
a federal public health insurance program primarily for the elderly and for patients with kidney disease

---

Medigap insurance
the informal name for insurance plans sold by private insurance companies to cover healthcare services/products that are not covered by Medicare

from private insurance companies. Additionally, many patients come to their physicians carrying advertisements for medications or procedures that they have seen on television, in magazines, or on the Internet. This pervasive marketing focused on the individual is highly effective. Individually focused health marketing has also been highly successful in the vitamin, supplement, and health equipment industries.

Effective and efficient health marketing endeavors must be delivered not only to individual consumers but also to physicians and health insurance companies. In the United States, most insured individuals are covered by one of two types of health insurance: public insurance, such as Medicare and **Medicaid**, or private insurance, which is most often purchased for patients and consumers by their employers. Because health insurance plays such a strong role in determining the kinds of health services people receive and the settings in which services are delivered, healthcare marketers must consider employers who choose health insurance plans for their employees, and even the government, as potential consumers of healthcare and ensure that they deliver effective marketing information to these entities. This topic is discussed in depth in the next chapter.

Medicaid
a joint state and federal public health insurance program for specific categories of the poor

CHAPTER QUESTIONS

1. What are the differences, both subtle and obvious, between being a patient and being a consumer of healthcare?
2. What does it mean to "shop" for healthcare? What makes shopping for healthcare difficult for most people? What would make it easier?
3. What advice would you offer to Matt in the case study at the beginning of this chapter?

CHAPTER EXERCISES

1. *Pharmaceuticals and the consumer*

   The media is saturated with advertisements for pharmaceuticals, both prescription and over the counter (OTC). However, sometimes the purpose of advertised medications is difficult to understand or unclear. Find two Internet, two print, and two television or radio advertisements for medications (either prescription or OTC), and analyze each on these points:

   ➤ What is the target market for the advertisement?

➤ What is the overarching message communicated by the advertisement?

➤ What assumptions is the advertisement based on?

➤ What specific information does the advertisement provide regarding costs, benefits, and side effects?

From your analysis, what conclusions can you draw about the individually focused pharmaceutical advertising directed at consumers?

2. *Medigap plans and the patient*

Your favorite aunt, Debbie, has just turned 65 and is now eligible for Medicare. She is fit and healthy and has no chronic illnesses. She knows you are an expert on healthcare, so she asks you to help her choose a Medigap plan to supplement her Medicare coverage. You sit down at a computer with her and type "Medigap" into the Internet browser.

➤ Describe the results of your Medigap search.

➤ Propose a logical, reasonable method or process for you and Aunt Debbie to use to shop for Medigap plans.

➤ Choose a plan.

Write a one-page paper describing how you felt while you were helping Aunt Debbie choose a Medigap plan.

REFERENCES

AlGhamdi, K. M., and N. A. Moussa. 2012. "Internet Use by the Public to Search for Health-Related Information." *International Journal of Health Informatics* 81 (6): 363–73.

Boulton, G. 2012. "Health Website Aimed at Latinos." *Milwaukee Journal Sentinel* April 13.

Kulick, D. L. 2013. "Coronary Artery Bypass Graft Surgery (CABG)." MedicineNet.com. www.medicinenet.com/coronary_artery_bypass_graft/article.htm.

Martin, A. B., D. Lassman, B. Washington, A. Catlin, and the National Health Expenditure Accounts Team. 2012. "Growth in US Health Spending Remained Slow in 2010: Health Share of Gross Domestic Product Was Unchanged from 2009." *Health Affairs* 31 (1): 208–19.

Toussaint, J. 2012. "Creating Healthcare Value." Studer Group Forum at the AUPHA Annual Meeting, Minneapolis, MN, June 2.

CHAPTER 7

PAYERS

After studying this chapter, you will be able to

➤ distinguish between public and private insurers and prospective versus retrospective reimbursement,

➤ identify the primary public insurers,

➤ list different insurance reimbursement mechanisms, and

➤ discuss payers as customers.

CASE STUDY: DEFINING PAYERS

"OK, everybody," the CEO said, "we need to start thinking seriously about our payer mix. I know that this recession has left lots of folks unemployed and without health insurance, but we need to figure out how to attract folks who do have insurance. And I don't mean public insurance. Yes, I know that the elderly are the fastest-growing segment in society, but Medicare is just not a good payer. And with so many people unemployed, our Medicaid and CHIP patient numbers are exploding. But they don't pay worth a darn either. Do you even know how much bad debt for uncompensated care the board wrote off last month? We have too many patients who can't pay for care themselves or have public insurance whose reimbursement barely covers our expenses. I know we can't turn poor people and the elderly away, but can't we discourage so many of them from showing up here? If we are ever going to get out of the red and into the black, we need to attract better payers."

The people around the table were trying to hide their yawns. They had heard this tirade before. In fact, they heard it at every meeting. But this time, attention was suddenly directed at Hassan Alsaad. He almost jumped when the CEO singled him out.

"Hassan, isn't this your area? I mean, isn't this what you marketing people are supposed to do—attract the right kind of patients so we can make money? We need patients with better insurance. Or even better, we need private-pay patients with lots of money who can buy expensive services. Why aren't you attracting those payers? Why are they going to other facilities? Why can't you get them to come here? I want you to go out and sign new contracts with insurance companies that reimburse at higher rates right now. Is that so hard? What are you and your people doing down there in marketing anyway?"

All eyes turned to Hassan. Working hard to keep his composure and not let panic set in, he said, "Sure, I'll get right on it." Thankfully, the focus of the meeting changed and attention was directed at someone else, and Hassan was able to collect his thoughts. Good grief! What was the big deal about payers? How in the world could he be expected to attract and influence a specific type of patient or a specific type of payer? He was an expert at informing the public about services and providers and attracting them to the facility, but he had never really thought about attracting specific patients with specific kinds of insurance or insurers themselves. Was it even ethical to do that?

PAYERS

In the United States, the entity paying for health services often is not the entity choosing the product or service or the entity receiving or using the service; unlike in other industries, the lines between buyers, sellers, and payers are blurred in healthcare. In the United States, private and public insurers, also called third-party payers, primarily pay for healthcare. In 2011, the major public (government) insurers—Medicare and Medicaid—accounted for 36 percent of all national health expenditures (NHE). Smaller government programs, including the Children's Health Insurance Program (CHIP), the Department of Defense, and the Department of Veterans Affairs, accounted for just under 4 percent. Private health insurance spending (including self-insured organizations) represented 33 percent, and out-of-pocket spending—payment for healthcare with one's own personal funds—made up 11 percent. Other third-party programs, such as maternal and child health, workers' compensation, and the Indian Health Service, represented a little over 7 percent (CMS 2012).

HEALTH INSURANCE IN THE UNITED STATES

private health insurers
non-government-owned, for-profit and not-for-profit private businesses that sell health insurance

As mentioned earlier, the two predominant forms of health insurance in the United States are (1) private and (2) public. **Private health insurers** are non-government-owned private businesses that sell health insurance. Private health insurance companies can be for-profit or not-for-profit. The basic difference between for-profit and not-for-profit companies is what they do with their profits—that is, money they earn over and above their expenses. In for-profit health insurance companies, profit can be distributed to owners or stockholders/shareholders or invested back in the organization. In not-for-profit health insurance organizations, profit must be reinvested in the organization, not distributed among its owners. It is a great misconception that not-for-profit health insurers don't earn profit; they do.

While all government-owned health insurers are not-for-profit by definition, it is another great misconception that all not-for-profit health insurance organizations are public or governmental organizations; they are not. Furthermore, not-for-profit and for-profit health insurers are taxed differently. Organizations cannot simply declare themselves to be not-for-profit; they must earn not-for-profit status by providing valuable services or public benefits to the community over and above the products and services they sell.

PRIVATE HEALTH INSURERS

tax-exempt status of health insurance
the federal provision that treats employer spending on employee health insurance as a tax-deductible business expense, not as taxable income

Private health insurance companies sell health insurance plans and policies primarily to individuals and to employers. Self-insured organizations also are considered private health insurers. Most people in the United States who have private health insurance receive it through their employer or are insured by their parents' or spouse's employer. The **tax-exempt status of health insurance** gives employers a financial incentive to provide health insurance for their workers in lieu of a portion of their wages; the money that employers spend on insurance for employees is treated as a tax-deductible business expense. Likewise, employees have a strong financial incentive to accept health insurance from their employer because they can pay their portion of the insurance cost with money that is not taxed. This two-way tax benefit explains why health insurance is so tightly bound to employment in the United States. While employees tend to view employer-paid health insurance as a gift additional to their pay, it is not. Health insurance is part of employees' compensation package; as stated earlier, a portion of employees' pretax cash wages is used to pay for their share of the insurance cost. While some employers pay the entire premium (i.e., cost) of their employees' insurance, employers typically contribute approximately 80 percent of the cost of the insurance and the employee funds the rest (Reinhardt 2009). In 2012, 61 percent of all firms offered their employees health benefits (Kaiser Family Foundation and Health Research & Educational Trust 2012, 4). Regardless of whether one's employer pays the entire premium or the cost of the premium is shared between the employer and the employee, the ability to pay for health insurance with pretax income is a valuable employment benefit.

Even when insured, patients are typically responsible for **out-of-pocket expenses**, which can amount to large sums of money. Most health insurance plans have deductibles and cost-sharing arrangements in the form of coinsurance and copayments. *Deductibles* are a flat, predetermined amount that the patient must pay before the insurance company begins to pay for care; once the patient has met the deductible, the insurance company will pay for care according to the policy's cost-sharing arrangement. *Coinsurance* is a predetermined division of costs that specifies what the patient's and the insurer's share of the bill will be once the patient meets the deductible. For example, in a 30/70 coinsurance arrangement, the patient will pay 30 percent of post-deductible costs and the insurance company will pay the remaining 70 percent. Being responsible for only 30 percent of one's bill may sound good, but many healthcare services are incredibly expensive; in 2005 the median cost of coronary artery bypass graft surgery was $25,140 (Neale 2010), 30 percent of which comes to $7,542.

Copayments, on the other hand, are predetermined fees for specific categories of services, regardless of the time, materials/supplies, or personnel involved in delivering the services. Copayments are similar to movie tickets: A theater offers tickets at a set price, regardless of whether the movie is a 90-minute comedy, a two-hour action film, or a two-and-a-half-hour epic. Likewise, a patient pays a predetermined copayment for brand-name prescriptions, generic prescriptions, primary care office visits, emergency room visits, and specialist visits, regardless of what the visit entails or what the medication is. Thus, even when insured employees use healthcare services, they still are payers because they are responsible for out-of-pocket expenses.

Many large employers offer their employees an array of health plans with different coverage, cost-sharing arrangements, and premiums. While employees are free to choose among the plans their employer has selected, they don't choose the individual benefits included in the plans. Hundreds of private insurance companies exist nationwide, most of which offer hundreds of different policies and plans, sometimes fine-tuned to employers' specifications. As when choosing a physician or a facility, employees have little data on which to base their choice of plan, so most select their plans according to price or recommendations from family and friends without understanding the coverage, cost-sharing, or quality details (Toussaint 2012). Family and friends may have experience with or heard stories about certain insurance

out-of-pocket expenses
non-premium expenses, such as deductibles, that patients must pay for with their own funds

companies, and employees' coworkers may have experience with or information about the plans offered by their employer. Health insurers, through their marketing and public relations efforts, may have a local or national reputation. By typing "choosing health insurance" into a search engine, employees can find at least a dozen websites offering advice, tips, and methods for choosing an insurer. All these factors play a part in an employee's choice of health plans.

Two important categories of private insurance are not purchased by employers. The first is health insurance purchased individually. Most employer-sponsored health plans are priced at a group rate, which in effect lowers the cost per person. It is rather like buying in bulk, and the savings are passed along to the employer. When an individual purchases an individual health insurance policy, he/she does not receive a discount. The insurer investigates the individual in great detail to determine his/her health risks, and the more risks the person has, the higher the premium. Health insurance is a business, and actuaries and underwriters must be careful not to underestimate the insurer's financial risk when writing a policy for an individual. In addition, they must consider *moral hazard*—the assumption that a person wouldn't be seeking to purchase health insurance if he/she didn't need it or intend to use it. Thus, individually purchased health insurance is prohibitively expensive for most people and is a small part of the health insurance market.

On the other hand, the second type of individually purchased private health insurance is a large, growing market. Medicare supplement plans, commonly called *Medigap plans*, are designed to cover services not covered by Medicare, including the "donut hole" in Medicare Part D prescription coverage, and in many cases also pay part or all of Medicare's deductibles and cost shares. Thousands of Medigap plans are offered by hundreds of private insurance companies. Some provide comprehensive coverage, while others cover only specific illnesses or situations. America's Health Insurance Plans, a national trade association representing the health insurance industry, reported that the number of seniors enrolled in Medigap coverage reached 9.8 million in 2011 and continues to increase (AHIP 2012). Given the increasing number of seniors in the United States, one can only expect this large segment of the private insurance market to steadily grow in upcoming years.

PUBLIC HEALTH INSURERS

public health insurers
not-for-profit insurance plans owned and run by the federal government or by the states; examples include Medicare, Medicaid, and CHIP

Medicare, Medicaid, CHIP, and the Veterans Administration are likely the largest and best-known **public health insurers**. In 2011, Medicare—the federal health insurance program primarily for the elderly—accounted for approximately 21 percent of NHE, and Medicaid—the state and federal cosponsored health insurance program for specific categories of the poor—accounted for 15 percent (CMS 2012). Medicare, Medicaid, and CHIP contract with providers, facilities, and health systems that agree to accept patients covered by these programs, to accept reimbursement rates set by the states for services provided to these patients, and to meet specific program requirements. As Medicare and Medicaid together make up approximately 36 percent of NHE, few health providers refuse these patients, despite that the programs' reimbursement rates are often lower than private insurers' reimbursement rates. Providers in traditional fee-for-service settings are not required to accept every Medicare, Medicaid, or CHIP patient who requests services. However, providers that have managed care or health maintenance organization (HMO) arrangements with these programs, such as Medicare+Choice and state Medicaid and CHIP managed care organizations (MCOs), must accept Medicare, Medicaid, and CHIP patients in compliance with their managed care contracts. Most Medicaid and CHIP beneficiaries nationwide are enrolled in some form of MCO (Gifford et al. 2011). Patients in Medicare, Medicaid, and CHIP MCOs often have free choice of providers within the MCO.

PAYMENT MECHANISMS

Traditionally, providers have been reimbursed on a **fee-for-service** basis by both private and public insurers. In a fee-for-service arrangement, providers create a comprehensive list of services they provided to a patient and the materials, supplies, and facilities they used to provide those services and then bill the patient's insurer (or the patient if he/she is self-pay) for each item on the list. The amount that insurers reimburse providers for a particular service is based on usual, customary, and reasonable (UCR) charges, which consider the provider's usual fee for the service, the fee that providers in general customarily charge for the service, and whether the amount requested by the provider is reasonable. UCR reimbursement is not a set fee but rather falls within an acceptable fee range or interval, and it is *retrospective*; providers don't know the exact amount they will be reimbursed for any service until after the service has been provided, been billed for, and passed UCR scrutiny (see Chapter 1). As providers steadily increased the reimbursements they requested for services, the UCR ranges for all services crept steadily upward.

In the early 1980s, public insurers became increasingly concerned about the rising costs of healthcare. After a few failed attempts at price controls, Medicare introduced Diagnosis-Related Groups (DRGs) for inpatient care in 1983. This system reimburses providers on the basis of a predetermined fee schedule for specific diagnoses. The amount of time, effort, and materials involved in the care and treatment of a patient does not matter; the provider is reimbursed only the preset amount for the patient's diagnosis. Payment based on DRGs is *prospective* because the provider knows the reimbursement amount before the service is provided (see Chapter 1). DRGs were a shock to most providers; before this system was implemented, few knew how much it actually cost to provide a service or treatment. Because DRGs are a preset fee schedule, it behooves providers to deliver services at costs that are lower than the DRG reimbursement amounts; otherwise, they would lose money on each patient.

fee-for-service
a retrospective reimbursement system in which providers create a comprehensive list of services they provided to a patient and the materials, supplies, and facilities they used to provide those services and then bill the patient's insurer (or the patient, if he/she is self-pay) for each item on the list

Shortly thereafter, Medicare introduced a prospective payment schedule for out-patient care called the Resource-Based Relative Value Scale (RBRVS). Under this system, reimbursement is calculated by multiplying the combined costs of providing a service (adjusted according to geographic location) by a conversion factor. It became clear early on that some procedures and treatments were money makers and some were money losers. Medicare, which had been a source of relatively easy money for providers, had become a tight-fisted, strict, careful insurer. For the first time, providers thought about how to attract and maintain a financially favorable **payer mix**.

payer mix
the combination of payers, including third parties and individuals, from which a healthcare organization is receiving reimbursement

HMOs also were a product of the early 1980s. As opposed to DRGs and RBRVS, HMOs initially were not about saving money; they were intended to revolutionize the delivery of healthcare by reversing all the perverse incentives driving the healthcare industry. Instead of waiting until people became sick and then trying to heal them, HMOs were supposed to deliver front-end care designed to help keep people healthy in the first place. Rather than having ill-informed healthcare consumers move from provider to provider and receive ineffective, duplicative care, HMOs assigned members to providers who orchestrated their care. HMO physicians did not automatically admit patients to hospitals for costly extensive testing, rehabilitation, and inpatient stays; they screened patients first to determine whether hospital care and expensive services and treatments were necessary. And most important, HMOs put physicians at financial risk for the care of their patients via per member per month reimbursement, whereas fee-for-service reimbursement created a financial incentive for physicians to provide more care to earn more money.

Early studies found that HMO members had better health outcomes than did traditional fee-for-service patients, and at a significantly lower cost. These early findings greatly impressed payers, and soon HMOs no longer were considered a new and different way to deliver care and reverse perverse incentives; they became the tool payers used to try to reduce healthcare costs. However, many physicians and patients came to despise the strictness of HMOs, and less restrictive arrangements, collectively called managed care, came into being. Along the continuum between fee-for-service and HMOs there are myriad insurance mechanisms, including prospective payment organizations and preferred provider organizations, that blend features of these two extremes.

COMPETING FOR PAYERS

Healthcare marketers need to focus on payers as customers. While attracting a large payer in the form of contracting with a large health system, insurer, or managed care organization is an important health marketing endeavor, there are important new marketing opportunities for attracting the business of individual self-pay patients. Because self-pay patients are not purchasing their care through an insurance plan, providers are under no restrictions as to how much to charge them for services. One example is the website

MediBid.com, which enables patients to deal directly with physicians to save money on self-pay care (Zoom Information, Inc. 2013):

> MediBid.com is the only company of its kind. Unlike the other guys, we don't refer you to a particular doctor or facility, we actually give you CHOICE. You choose the doctor or medical facility that is right for YOU. You create a request describing the medical procedure you need, no matter how big or small, and doctors and facilities from all over the country and the world Bid on your request. We let the doctors come to you. They Bid upfront, cash prices, and you choose the doctor that is right for you based not only on the price, but on their location, credentials, accommodations, etc. Once you accept a doctor's bid, the entire relationship is directly between you and your doctor, as it should be. Here at MediBid, we value patient privacy, freedom of choice, access, and transparency.

Another opportunity to attract individual patients is presented by **medical tourism**. At a time when even insured patients experience "sticker shock" upon learning the out-of-pocket costs they must pay for expensive health services here in the United States, many US residents are seeking less expensive yet safe, high-quality care in hospitals abroad. "High costs and long waiting lists at home, new technology and skills in destination countries alongside reduced transport costs and Internet marketing have all played a role" (Connell 2006, 1093). According to the Medical Tourism Association, cost savings can amount to up to 90 percent (MTA 2013). Through individualized, Internet-based marketing, health systems and providers abroad have found a way to inform and attract patients from all over the world.

medical tourism
traveling to other countries to obtain less expensive yet safe, high-quality care

CONCLUSION

Ultimately, everyone pays for healthcare. Insurers pay for it, employers pay for it, and the government pays for it, but individuals pay for it, too, whether out of pocket, through taxes, through their employers, or through their insurance. Exactly who the payer is and what the payer is paying for can be difficult to identify in healthcare. Other chapters in this book argue that healthcare marketers need to inform and attract patients, physicians, facilities, and health systems. This chapter adds to this list, arguing that healthcare marketers need to inform and attract payers: individual patients, employers, health insurers, and even the government. Because the market for healthcare services in the United States is so complex and convoluted, healthcare marketers must not only deeply understand how to inform, communicate with, attract, and meet the needs of patients, physicians, and payers but also have a clear and current understanding of the US healthcare system.

CHAPTER QUESTIONS

1. What are the major differences between public and private insurers?
2. What has been the overall impact of making health insurance exempt from taxes?
3. What is payer mix, and what is its role in healthcare marketing?
4. What is medical tourism, and why would a healthcare marketer be interested in it?

CHAPTER EXERCISES

1. *Identifying payers*

   In this chapter's case study, Hassan is told to change his approach to marketing by attracting payers in addition to providing information about services and attracting physicians. Payer mix is an important concept in healthcare. Hassan asks himself whether it is ethical for marketers to try to attract generous payers and discourage those that are not so generous. What do you think?

2. *Benefits of tax-exempt status*

   The tax-exempt status of health insurance is a great incentive for employers and employees to purchase employment-based health insurance. Assume that you earn $1,000 and pay $20 for health insurance per pay period and that your tax rate is 10 percent. Create two scenarios, one in which you pay for the insurance before your wages are taxed and one in which you pay for the insurance after your wages are taxed.

   ➤ What is the difference in your net pay?

   ➤ What is the difference in the tax you pay?

   ➤ How do these differences impact the amount of tax revenue collected by the federal government?

3. *What is your opinion on tax subsidies of employer-based health insurance?*

   Exercise #2 shows that employer-sponsored health insurance is highly subsidized by the federal government. On one hand, health insurance is a public good that enhances the health and well-being of US residents and thereby promotes economic productivity. On the other hand, the tax revenue lost by the federal government could ease the US budget deficit. Where do you stand on this issue?

REFERENCES

America's Health Insurance Plans (AHIP). 2012. "Nine Out of Ten Seniors Satisfied with Their Medigap Coverage." www.ahip.org/News/Press-Room/2012/Nine-out-of-Ten-Seniors-Satisfied-with-their-Medigap-Coverage.aspx.

Centers for Medicare & Medicaid Services (CMS). 2012. "Table 4: National Health Expenditures by Source of Funds and Type of Expenditures: Calendar Years 2005–2011." www.cms.gov/Research-Statistics-Data-and-Systems/Statistics-Trends-and-Reports/NationalHealthExpendData/Downloads/tables.pdf.

Connell, J. 2006. "Medical Tourism: Sea, Sun, Sand, and Surgery." *Tourism Management* 27: 1093–100.

Gifford, K., V. K. Smith, D. Snipes, and J. Paradise. 2011. "A Profile of Medicaid Managed Care Programs in 2010: Findings from a 50-State Survey." Washington, DC: Kaiser Commission on Medicaid and the Uninsured. Published in September. http://kaiserfamilyfoundation.files.wordpress.com/2013/01/8220.pdf.

Kaiser Family Foundation and Health Research & Educational Trust. 2012. "Employer Health Benefits: 2012 Summary of Findings." http://kaiserfamilyfoundation.files.wordpress.com/2013/03/8346-employer-health-benefits-annual-survey-summary-of-findings-0912.pdf.

Medical Tourism Association (MTA). 2013. "Medical Tourism FAQs." www.medicaltourismassociation.com/en/medical-tourism-faq-s.html.

Neale, T. 2010. "CABG Cost May Be Related to Procedure Volume." *MedPage Today* July 26. www.medpagetoday.com/Cardiology/Atherosclerosis/21390.

Reinhardt, U. 2009. "Is Employer-Based Health Insurance Worth Saving? *New York Times* May 22. http://economix.blogs.nytimes.com/2009/05/22/is-employer-based-health-insurance-worth-saving/.

Toussaint, J. 2012. "Creating Healthcare Value." Studer Group Forum at the 2012 AUPHA Annual Meeting, Minneapolis, MN, June 2.

Zoom Information, Inc. 2013. MediBid Inc. company profile. www.zoominfo.com/c/Medibid-Inc/347582692.

CHAPTER 8

THE PUBLIC

After studying this chapter, you will be able to

➤ explain the concept of community benefits,

➤ illustrate the concept of public health,

➤ define health literacy,

➤ describe health promotion,

➤ apply social marketing to public health situations, and

➤ evaluate the role of the healthcare marketer in relation to public health.

CASE STUDY: FIRST LADY MICHELLE OBAMA AND *LET'S MOVE!*

Mary Elizabeth LeMont, media specialist, and her boss, Juanita Santos, public relations coordinator, worked in the Office of Marketing and Public Relations at Grannus Medical. They just attended a meeting of Grannus's board, where they presented a proposal that Grannus Medical participate in First Lady Michelle Obama's *Let's Move!* campaign. The proposal was well received. Both Mary Elizabeth and Juanita were impressed with the First Lady's initiative to try to end childhood obesity within a generation's time, and they knew that this type of campaign fit well with Grannus and its commitment to enhance quality of life among the communities and people it served.

Located in the eastern region of North Carolina, Grannus Medical's eight hospitals served more than 2.5 million people from more than 20 counties. As part of Grannus Medical's goal to enhance quality of life, it engaged in initiatives to better serve the surrounding communities and increase health awareness. Some of its efforts included providing healthcare without reimbursement (charity care), offering healthcare programs to the community at no charge, and non-healthcare initiatives that addressed broader community issues. In fiscal year 2011–2012, Grannus offered more than $130 million in **community benefit** activities and services (see Exhibit 8.1 for a breakdown of the distribution of funds to various efforts).

If approved by the board, the *Let's Move!* initiative at Grannus would be categorized as a community health improvement service (which represented 16 percent of the

community benefits
activities, programs, and healthcare provided to promote and enhance quality of life among the community at large

EXHIBIT 8.1
Breakdown of Fund Distribution to Grannus Medical's Community Benefit Efforts, Fiscal Year 2011–2012

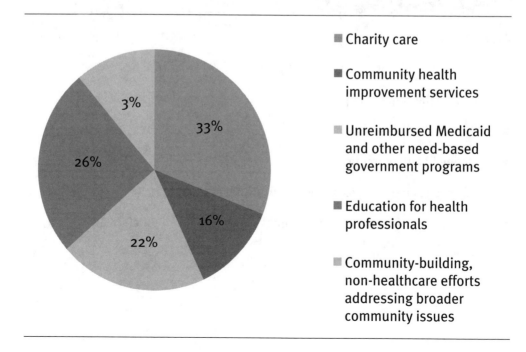

- Charity care
- Community health improvement services
- Unreimbursed Medicaid and other need-based government programs
- Education for health professionals
- Community-building, non-healthcare efforts addressing broader community issues

community benefits provided in 2011–2012) and could potentially reach more than 2.5 million people.

Launched in February 2010, *Let's Move!* had a simple goal. As stated by former US Surgeon General Regina Benjamin, "The goal of this initiative is solving the problem of childhood obesity in a generation, so that kids born today will grow up healthier and be better able to pursue their dreams" (HHS 2011). To this end, *Let's Move!* focused on encouraging food outlets to offer healthy choices, supporting legislation that funds healthy school lunches, increasing access to healthy food choices, and inspiring people to move for at least 60 minutes per day. Mrs. Obama became a highly visible spokesperson for the program via popular media, including talk shows such as *The Ellen DeGeneres Show* and *Late Night with Jimmy Fallon*. She also attended schools and exercised with students and planted a vegetable garden on the White House lawn. All of her *Let's Move!* activities centered on supporting healthy living. She used humor and encouragement to direct attention to the issue of childhood obesity in the United States and offered ways to effectively address the problem.

In addition to the promotional efforts by Mrs. Obama, commitments were secured from Walmart and Disney. Walmart pledged to make its food offerings healthier and more affordable (CNN 2011), and Disney changed its food advertising policy. By 2015, Disney's television and radio channels would market only foods that met its nutrition guidelines, which promoted consumption of fruits and vegetables and limited intake of calories, sugar, sodium, and saturated fat (*Let's Move!* 2012).

Let's Move! also offered tool kits, such as *Let's Move Faith and Communities*, *Let's Move Outside*, and *Chefs Move! to Schools*, as well as *Let's Move!* for healthcare providers (see www.letsmove.gov/health-care-providers). The healthcare initiative encouraged providers to take five steps (*Let's Move!* 2013):

1. Join *Let's Move!*
2. Measure patients' body mass index (BMI), and counsel patients about the benefits of exercise and good diets.
3. Talk with patients about breast-feeding and first foods for infants.
4. Share the 5210 "prescription" for healthier living: per day, eat 5 fruits and vegetables, limit television and video games to no more than 2 hours, do 1 hour of exercise, and drink 0 sugar-sweetened drinks.
5. Serve as leaders in their communities by sharing their knowledge of healthy behavior with the public.

Mary Elizabeth and Juanita's proposal focused on *Let's Move!* for healthcare providers. If the proposal were approved, Grannus's dietitians would be scheduled to team up with local farmers to provide nutritional information to local schools about the fruits and vegetables grown in the schools' gardens. Its allied health professionals would measure school children's BMI (with parental permission) with the BMI percentage calculator for children and teens (see http://apps.nccd.cdc.gov/dnpabmi/) as well as explain what BMI was and why it mattered. Finally, Grannus's marketing team (Mary Elizabeth and Juanita) would direct the production of marketing materials about healthy eating and exercise ideas for children for distribution to pediatricians and general practitioners who had privileges at any of Grannus's medical facilities in the 20-county region.

The impact Grannus could have as a partner in the *Let's Move!* campaign could not be overstated. The consequences of childhood obesity included high blood pressure and high cholesterol, which were risk factors for heart disease, type 2 diabetes, joint problems, sleep apnea, and asthma (see www.cdc.gov/obesity/childhood/basics.html). In eastern North Carolina, about 30 percent of children were considered obese. This percentage was almost twice as high as the national average of 17 percent (Pediatric Healthy Weight Research and Treatment Center 2013).

HEALTHCARE MARKETING, PUBLIC HEALTH, AND SOCIAL MARKETING

Marketing and public health might seem to be an odd match. *Public health* consists of civic activities, laws, and regulations designed to protect the health and well-being of all citizens. Campaigns such as *Let's Move!* are one type of public health initiative.

Marketing, on the other hand, is usually considered to be the activities and techniques used to promote and sell products or services. In the case study, Mary Elizabeth and Juanita work in the Office of Marketing and Public Relations at Grannus Medical, but for the *Let's Move!* campaign, they will be engaged in social marketing, which uses the foundations and basics of marketing to influence the health and wellness behaviors of individuals and groups. To understand social marketing and how it fits with marketing and public health, let us first explore the concepts of public health, health literacy, and health promotion.

PUBLIC HEALTH

public health
civic activities, laws, and regulations designed to protect the health and well-being of a population

A 1988 study conducted by the Institute of Medicine (IOM) defined the mission of **public health** as "the fulfillment of society's interest in assuring the conditions in which people can be healthy." The study went on to explain that public health is the "organized community effort aimed at the prevention of disease and the promotion of health" (IOM Committee for the Study of the Future of Public Health 1988, 40–41). One can better understand the concept of public health by contrasting it with medical care. Medical care is a one-on-one interaction between a healthcare provider or caregiver and a patient. For the most part, the provider focuses on one person at a time. He does what he can to enhance that one person's health and then moves on to the next person. Most people are familiar with this healthcare process.

Public health, on the other hand, aims to enhance the health and well-being of a group or a population, not an individual. For example, *Let's Move!* focuses on children, not on one particular child. Public health endeavors work best when many people engage in them. For instance, when one person decides not to smoke inside a restaurant but many other people do, that person's actions benefit his/her own health (perhaps with questionable results, due to secondhand smoke). However, when no one smokes in the restaurant, everyone's health benefits. Thus, antismoking laws work to everyone's benefit and, to paraphrase the IOM study mentioned earlier, create an environment in which everyone can be healthier.

Over the twentieth century, the average life expectancy of Americans increased from 45 to 75 years. Public health endeavors have contributed more to Americans' improved health and well-being than has medical care (Schneider 2004, 7):

> Only 5 of those additional 30 years can be attributed to medical care itself. The majority of the gain has come from improvements in public health, broadly defined to include better nutrition, housing, sanitation, and occupational safety.

Public health pervades nearly every aspect of our daily lives, and its scope is wide. For example, the laws that ensure eating establishments keep cold food cold enough and hot food hot enough are public health regulations. The antismoking laws mentioned earlier and the health warnings on tobacco packaging are public health initiatives. The rules governing seat belt and safety helmet use and blood alcohol levels for drivers are public health regulations. The push to increase hand washing to prevent the spread of colds and the flu is a public health endeavor. The famous "brain on drugs" egg in the hot frying pan is a public health advertisement, as are antilittering, clean air and water, and recycling campaigns.

Public health is an enigma. It is vitally important, widely unrecognized, and often contentious and controversial. It also is hard to measure. While a coronary unit in a hospital might accurately cite the number of deaths that have been averted as a result of coronary bypass procedures, how can one accurately measure the number of deaths averted by the use of car seats, seat belt laws, or antismoking regulations? Public health is not as tangible as cutting-edge, lifesaving medical procedures and technology. Public health initiatives can, however, be shocking and upsetting. For example, in response to the large number of babies who have been smothered while sleeping with adults, a recent advertisement in Milwaukee, Wisconsin, depicted a baby sleeping in an adult bed with a butcher knife and asserted that a baby sleeping with an adult in an adult bed is as endangered as a baby sleeping with a knife. Finally, public health often infringes on private, sensitive issues, such as the use of birth control and the prevention of HIV/AIDS and other sexually transmitted diseases.

More challenging, however, is the fact that public health asks everyone to give up some of their personal freedom for the good of society. *Let's Move!* asks parents to improve their diet and exercise routines on behalf of their children, smokers are asked not to smoke, drivers are asked to wear seat belts, and individuals are encouraged to get vaccinations. In today's world it might be hard to imagine why anyone would not want to properly dispose of human waste or live in a community that did not ensure the proper treatment of drinking water, but each of these public health endeavors was controversial in its time. So the legitimate marketing question is, how can the individual be influenced and persuaded to give up conveniences and adopt personal behaviors that enhance the health and well-being of many?

Actually, the pertinent questions might not be how to influence health behaviors but rather whether laws and regulations should infringe on individual rights for the benefit of the collective. In a capitalist market society, how much personal sacrifice, inconvenience, and even freedom should be expected or demanded of individuals for the benefit of the public? How do we know that the sacrifices and inconveniences are effective and worthwhile? For instance, how do we know if *Let's Move!* is successful? How do we define its worth? Should a free society force citizens to engage in health behaviors for their own good? Shouldn't free people be allowed to do unhealthy or even dangerous things if they want to? All these questions point to a common debate: Is using the persuasive techniques and processes of marketing to influence health behaviors and beliefs a reasonable and ethical endeavor?

HEALTH LITERACY

health literacy
the degree to which one has and understands health information essential to making informed health decisions

Healthy People 2010 (see Chapter 2) identified **health literacy** as a fundamental component of US society's health. It defined *health literacy* as "the degree to which individuals have the capacity to obtain, process, and understand basic health information needed to make appropriate health decisions" (HHS 2010).

Health literacy is far more than the ability to understand written materials; it also means having analytical and decision-making skills and the ability to apply those skills in health situations (HHS 2010). In most cases, societal questions regarding the rights of the individual versus the good of the many are addressed on the basis of two questions. First, does the unhealthy or dangerous activity impact someone other than the person carrying out the activity? Second, does the person carrying out the activity know the full impact of his/her actions, regardless of who is or is not in jeopardy? With regard to *Let's Move!*, for example, children themselves might not comprehend the danger posed by overweight and obesity, but overweight and obesity do impact their health as well as the health of the community. Children who are overweight are more likely to become overweight adults, and overweight/obesity in adulthood causes more health problems. Adults with health problems tend to lose income from decreased productivity in the workplace and increased absenteeism. Cost is another societal factor. In 2008, the medical care costs associated with obesity in the United States totaled approximately $147 billion (CDC 2012).

Another example illustrating this dichotomy in US society today is the controversy over vaccinations. Most public school systems require that children be vaccinated against common childhood diseases before they enter school, but there is a growing fear among some parents that these immunizations might cause more injury than good; the vaccination rate among children is lower than it has ever been since vaccinations became routine. This dissension is truly a health literacy issue. The World Health Organization (WHO 2010) lists six common misconceptions and falsehoods about immunizations:

1. Diseases had already begun to disappear before vaccines were introduced because of better hygiene and sanitation.

2. The majority of people affected by disease have been vaccinated.

3. The number of adverse events and deaths associated with "hot lots" of vaccine is greater than that associated with other batches. Parents should find the serial numbers of these lots and ensure their children are not inoculated with vaccines from this stock.

4. Vaccines cause many harmful side effects, illnesses, and even death, not to mention possible long-term effects that are not yet known.

5. Vaccine-preventable diseases have been virtually eliminated, so there is no need for children to be vaccinated.

6. Giving a child multiple vaccinations for different diseases at the same time increases the risk of harmful side effects and can overload the immune system.

These six assertions are scientifically false, yet they are regularly presented and discussed by the popular media as sound arguments. How can the average parent trying to ensure the health and well-being of his/her child know what to believe and what not to believe? The crux of such questions is health literacy.

What does health literacy have to do with marketing? As our vaccination example demonstrates, an overabundance of factually inaccurate health information circulates in society. While people have a basic right to believe or not believe whatever they want, how does erroneous health information become a common understanding? Health and wellness are emotional issues and can become explosive topics, particularly if one is personally affected. In addition, health information is technical and difficult to understand, especially for those who do not understand science. Finally, as is the case in all science, the results of early studies are often inconclusive, limited in scope, or conflicting, yet the media reports the results as definitive. This combination of emotion, risk, complexity, and heavy-handed reporting sets the stage for confusion and frustration among consumers and opens the door to the spread and acceptance of answers that are easier to understand and seem to make sense.

The dissemination of health information, whether by word of mouth, printed media, or electronic media (e.g., television or the Internet), is a form of marketing. If false information can be spread through the use of basic marketing techniques, so can the truth. Whether for the benefit of the individual or for the benefit of society, people need to hear accurate health information presented in a clear, persuasive, and understandable way to be able to make sound health decisions.

HEALTH PROMOTION AND SOCIAL MARKETING

Health promotion and social marketing are two sides of the same coin. **Health promotion** consists of activities designed to influence individual behaviors; health-related **social marketing**, on the other hand, is a concerted effort to influence groups, communities, or society as a whole. Both are centered on public health. For instance, Mrs. Obama's public appearances on talk shows and at school and sports events aim to raise individual awareness of the importance of healthy eating and exercise. The partnerships with Disney and Walmart and the development of a tool kit for healthcare providers are concentrated efforts to influence communities. The behavior of the individual impacts the community, and vice versa; as individuals engage in healthy behaviors, the community benefits, and as the community becomes healthier, the individuals in it benefit.

Social marketing often does not focus directly on health behaviors. In its broadest sense, the domain of social marketing is the betterment of all aspects of society. In this regard it can be a dynamic tool for instituting social change. Widespread public health advertisements are perhaps the most visible form of social marketing.

Some worthwhile campaigns have been less successful than hoped; while right-headed and well-meaning, the public health advertisements and campaigns of the past often failed because they did not adhere to the basic tenets of marketing. The belief seemed to be that just getting the information "out there" would be enough to change behavior and society. The thinking of the past runs along these lines: "If people just knew how dangerous an activity is, no intelligent person would ever engage in it." While this theory appears to be true and is emotionally appealing, people do not necessarily behave that way in the real world. It ignores the complexity of human behavior. In the case of smoking, for example, it does not address the myriad reasons, times, and places people smoke tobacco.

Many of the public health antilitter campaigns in the 1970s failed because they did not use the basic tools of marketing. They made no case for the personal benefits of not littering, offered no sense of personal efficacy/satisfaction for the nonlitterer (cleanup is a

health promotion
activities designed to influence individual behaviors that affect personal health

social marketing
the creation, communication, and delivery of information, events, programs, and so forth to influence individual behavior for the benefit of not only the individual but also the community and for the common good

collective effort and cannot be achieved through the efforts of one person alone), ignored the inconvenience of putting litter in trash containers, and were not tailored to target audiences (Kotler and Roberto 1989, 12). These campaigns ignored the basic marketing tenets of focusing on the consumer, conducting market research, and creating a systematic process for developing the marketing program (Weinreich 1999).

One key element of successful social marketing is to start with target markets that are "ready for action" (Kotler, Roberto, and Lee 2002, 53). In the case of *Let's Move!*, Mrs. Obama started by targeting children and parents; during one radio interview, she stated (Obama 2012):

> So the hope is that by starting the conversation with our children, you know, I find that adults are more inclined to make the changes for their kids more quickly than they will for themselves, and I've seen that happening across the country as we've begun this conversation.

Social marketing experts hold that it is harder to convince people to change their behaviors and beliefs than it is to convince them to try a new product. As mentioned earlier, public health efforts often target people's most personal behaviors and private, closely held beliefs. The price of changing behaviors and beliefs often is not monetary; rather, price represents time, effort, comfort, energy, opportunity costs, personal reputation, group membership, and even one's self-perception.

Social marketing has a branding problem; it has too many definitions, lacks clarity, and seems manipulative, and it is hard to measure and document its successes and failures (Andreasen 2006, 216). The lack of appreciation for social marketing at the top levels of health organizations is typified by the words of John Wanamaker, pioneer of the department store concept: "I know half the money I spend on advertising is wasted, but I can never find out which half" (Powell, Groves, and Dimos 2011, 8).

Some argue that instead of focusing on "downstream" behaviors and beliefs, social marketers should focus on the "upstream" causes of the behaviors and beliefs. For example, instead of trying to change smokers, social marketing should use the techniques and processes of marketing and focus on the social and physical determinants of smoking instead (Andreasen 2006, 7). Or instead of trying to change individuals' eating habits, social marketing should focus on the factors that encourage the habits (e.g., Walmart's initiative to make healthy foods affordable and accessible).

HEALTHCARE MARKETERS AS CRITICAL THINKERS AND CREATIVE PROBLEM SOLVERS

A strong case can be made for the role of healthcare marketers and the application of the marketing principles, techniques, and practices discussed in this book to social health and wellness betterment endeavors. Marketing is more than selling to the public. Because of the difficulties of influencing behaviors and beliefs, marketing health and wellness for individuals, groups, communities, and society is far more complex than simply providing information or applying the four generic Ps of product, price, place, and promotion. Social marketing has the potential to greatly enhance the health and well-being of the public—individuals, communities, and society.

CHAPTER QUESTIONS

1. What are the core differences between public health endeavors and traditional medical care delivery?
2. Gun violence is a pressing public health problem; gun control is a highly controversial public health proposal. Identify the key arguments for and against gun control solely from a public health perspective.
3. Select a timely social marketing topic and create a comprehensive list of its "prices" to individuals.

CHAPTER EXERCISES

1. *Something has to change, but what?*

   On New Year's Day, Pat finally summoned the nerve to step on the bathroom scale. Having a specific highest-possible weight in mind, Pat was distressed to find that she was heavier than she had expected. She knew something clearly needed to change, but what? After asking friends for advice, Pat had a long list of suggestions. Her friends recommended that she count calories, join one of the many weight loss clubs/organizations advertised nonstop on television and radio, join a gym, find a walking partner, start running, go on the grapefruit diet, stop eating all carbohydrates, eat more protein, eat breakfast and/or lunch, skip breakfast and/or lunch, never go out to eat again, give up pizza, stop eating chocolate, park two blocks away from all destinations, purchase weight loss/energy pills advertised in magazines, buy a treadmill and barbells—the list went on. The options were confusing, contradictory, and overwhelming, and many were expensive. From past experience, Pat knows that trying too many things at once never works.

How should Pat decide what to do? Create a list of five things Pat could do (or stop doing) to lose weight. Describe ways in which Pat can ascertain how effective each change will be. What sources or experts should she consult?

2. *You be on the board of Grannus*

Refer to the case study at the beginning of this chapter. If you were on the board, what would you think of the *Let's Move!* initiative? Would you support its implementation in eastern North Carolina? Why or why not?

Peruse the Internet for YouTube videos and news reports regarding *Let's Move!*. How would you evaluate the initiative to date? Consider, for example, the assertions made earlier in this chapter that the public health antilitter campaigns failed because they did not use the basic tools of marketing: They made no case for the personal benefits of not littering, offered no sense of personal efficacy/ satisfaction for the nonlitterer, ignored the inconvenience of putting litter in trash containers, and were not tailored to target audiences. Do you think Mrs. Obama's efforts and the *Let's Move!* campaign made a case for the personal benefits of healthy living? Do they offer a sense of personal efficacy/satisfaction for the "mover"? Have commitments been made to make eating healthier and exercising more accessible (more convenient)? Were efforts tailored to specific audiences? Did they start with target markets that were "ready for action"?

3. *The Affordable Care Act and the "Healthcare Updates" column*

You are an intern in the local community hospital's marketing and public relations department. The hospital employs about 500 people, and your department is responsible for publishing the monthly employee newsletter, *Insights*. The main purpose of the newsletter is to keep employees informed about hospital policies and to discuss subjects that might be of interest to them. Last month in the "News You Can Use" column, the hospital's human resources director wrote about preparing for retirement wisely; in the "Employee Health" column, one of the dietitians shared plant-based recipes for healthy living; and in the "Healthcare Updates" column, the CEO explained that the hospital's administrators had decided to adopt a new electronic health record system because it would help organize patient data and identify aspects of patient care that have worked well and improved quality in alignment with the expectations of the Affordable Care Act (ACA). The chief information officer (CIO) also contributed to the column, citing the time frame for training and implementation of the new system.

The CIO's column generated more comments and questions than your supervisor, Julia, had ever seen in her tenure at the hospital. Employees asked Julia about the ACA. One employee wrote in an e-mail, "I know it is complicated; can you help me understand the basics? Perhaps a series of columns about the ACA would be an idea for *Insights*." Another employee wrote, "How is the ACA going to affect my health insurance?" Still another wrote, "What does an electronic health record have to do with the ACA?" One employee called and asked, "What is this ACA, and what does it have to do with healthcare?"

Your supervisor brought the messages to your attention and asked you to write a draft for next month's "Healthcare Updates" column. She said, "I want you to write up an executive summary about the ACA. In two pages, double spaced, tell me what I would need to know about the basic tenets of the act. If you get on a roll, go ahead and write a two-page response to each of the questions I received."

You are a bit daunted. You know some details of the ACA, but you are by no means an expert on the subject. Using the following information and other references you may find, write one of the two-page answers Julia has asked you to compose.

The Patient Protection and Affordable Care Act (PPACA), also known as the *Affordable Care Act (ACA), Obamacare*, and *Obamacares*, was signed into law in March 2010. While the law is complex, the basic tenet of the law is to expand access to healthcare for US citizens and legal immigrants by increasing access to insurance coverage. The law addresses four basic areas:

1. *Coverage and access*

    a. Expanding access to health insurance coverage:

    In 2011, about 48.6 million people in the United States (15.7 percent of the population) did not have health insurance (US Census Bureau 2012). The

ACA expands coverage by requiring most US citizens and legal immigrants to have health insurance. If individuals refuse to purchase insurance, they pay a fine via a tax penalty. Individuals may obtain insurance via employment or health exchanges. Health exchanges will be established by the state or federal government. Via the exchanges, people may compare different insurance plan options and select a plan appropriate for themselves.

Businesses that employ 50 or more full-time employees are required to offer health insurance coverage; businesses that employ more than 200 employees must enroll employees in the employer-based health insurance plan unless an employee chooses not to be enrolled.

b. Expanding healthcare access for the poor through Medicaid expansion: Prior to implementation of the ACA, Medicaid covered only certain categories of persons. Low-income, childless, nondisabled, non-elderly adults did not qualify. In 2012, the US Supreme Court ruled that states may or may not expand Medicaid. However, even if a state decides not to expand Medicaid, low-income, childless, nondisabled, non-elderly adults will not qualify for subsidies by the state's health benefits exchange.

2. *Overall population health status*

According to WHO (2013), as of 2011 the United States ranked 34th among WHO member countries in terms of life expectancy of both sexes at birth. The following table compares life expectancies (in years) for men and women in the United States with life expectancies in Western European countries as of 2011.

Country	Men	Women
Italy	80	85
Canada	80	84
France	78	85
Germany	78	83
United Kingdom	79	82
United States	76	81

Source: Data from WHO (2013).

The ACA focuses on prevention, wellness, and public health activities via awards of grant money. Priority areas include health promotion; disease prevention; campaigns to promote exercise and better nutrition and life-styles (e.g., stop or do not start smoking cigarettes); maternal, infant, and early childhood health (e.g., home visits); teenage pregnancy and teen parenting skills; and pregnancy prevention.

3. *Quality*

In its 2000 report *To Err Is Human*, IOM disclosed that between 44,000 and 98,000 Americans die every year as a result of medical errors (Kohn, Corrigan, and Donaldson 2000). The ACA charges the US Department of Health and Human Services secretary with directing and creating a national strategy to improve the quality of patient care (including reduction of medical errors). To this end, funding focuses on areas such as comparative effectiveness research (e.g., the effect of hand washing on transmission of infections between caregivers and patients), development of quality measures to track improvements, and creation of a forum for publication of data pertaining to quality.

4. *Cost*

According to the Organisation for Economic Co-operation and Development (OECD 2011), people in the United States spend more money on healthcare than people in other countries do but benefit less from their expenditures. The United States spends about $2,830 per capita on ambulatory care (care provided by physicians, dentists, and so forth), which is 238 percent more than the average spending per capita on ambulatory care among Switzerland ($1,626), Canada ($1,171), Germany ($1,254), France ($1,062), and Japan ($787).

New models of care, including accountable care organizations (ACOs) and patient-centered medical homes (PCMHs), may improve the delivery of healthcare and contain costs. ACOs are characterized by a payment and healthcare delivery system that ties provider reimbursement to quality of care and reduced costs. PCMHs are designed to provide comprehensive primary care for patients throughout their lives. Patients have a "medical home" where interdisciplinary teams of healthcare providers provide coordinated care so that patient information is stored at one site. The importance of electronic health records (EHRs) in the delivery of coordinated care cannot be overstated. EHRs store information about each service provided to a patient so that all providers know what other providers have done on behalf of that patient.

The following sources provide more information on the topics highlighted here:

➤ *Basics of healthcare reform:* Kaiser Family Foundation (www.kff.org)

➤ *Insurance coverage in the United States:* US Census Bureau (www.census.gov)

➤ *Statistics comparing the United States and other countries:* World Health Organization (www.who.int)

➤ *Reducing medical errors to improve patient quality:* www.kaiseredu.org

➤ *ACOs:* www.healthcare.gov

➤ *PCMHs:* Agency for Healthcare Research and Quality PCMH Resource Center (www.pcmh.ahrq.gov)

REFERENCES

Andreasen, A. R. 2006. *Social Marketing in the 21st Century*. Thousand Oaks, CA: Sage Publications.

Centers for Disease Control and Prevention (CDC). 2012. "Overweight and Obesity: Causes and Consequences." Page updated April 27. www.cdc.gov/obesity/adult/causes/index .html.

CNN. 2011. "Walmart Joins Michelle Obama's *Let's Move!* Campaign." Eatocracy [blog]. Posted January 20. http://eatocracy.cnn.com/2011/01/20/walmart-joins-michelle-obamas-lets-move-campaign/.

Institute of Medicine (IOM) Committee for the Study of the Future of Public Health. 1988. *The Future of Public Health*. Washington, DC: National Academies Press.

Kohn, L. T., J. M. Corrigan, and M. S. Donaldson (eds.). 2000. *To Err Is Human: Building a Safer Health System*. Washington, DC: National Academies Press.

Kotler, P., and E. L. Roberto. 1989. *Social Marketing: Strategies for Changing Public Behavior*. New York: Free Press.

Kotler, P., N. Roberto, and N. R. Lee. 2002. *Social Marketing: Improving the Quality of Life*, second edition. Thousand Oaks, CA: Sage Publications.

Let's Move!. 2013. "5 Simple Steps to Success for Health Care Providers." www.letsmove.gov /health-care-providers.

———. 2012. "Today the First Lady Announces Disney's Healthy Food Marketing Standards." *Let's Move!* [blog]. Posted June 5. www.letsmove.gov/blog/2012/06/05 /today-first-lady-announces-disney%E2%80%99s-healthy-food-marketing-standards.

Obama, M. 2012. "First Lady: Nation's Health 'Starts with Our Kids.'" Interview by N. Conan, *Talk of the Nation*, NPR, June 12. www.npr.org/templates/transcript/transcript.php?storyId= 154854113.

Organisation for Economic Co-operation and Development (OECD). 2011. "Why Is Health Spending in the United States So High?" www.oecd.org/unitedstates/49084355.pdf.

Pediatric Healthy Weight Research and Treatment Center. 2013. "About Us: Background." Greenville, NC: East Carolina University Brody School of Medicine, Department of Pediatrics. www.ecu.edu/cs-dhs/pedsweightcenter/about.cfm.

Powell, G., S. Groves, and J. Dimos. 2011. *ROI of Social Media: How to Improve the Return on Your Social Marketing Investment*. Singapore: John Wiley & Sons (Asia) Pte. Ltd.

Schneider, M. 2004. *Introduction to Public Health*. Sudbury, MA: Jones and Bartlett.

US Census Bureau. 2012. "Health Insurance: Highlights: 2011." Page updated September 12. www.census.gov/hhes/www/hlthins/data/incpovhlth/2011/highlights.html.

US Department of Health and Human Services (HHS). 2011. "New York City Celebrates *Let's Move!* One Year Anniversary." News release, February 8. www.hhs.gov/news/press /2011pres/02/20110208a.html.

———. 2010. *Healthy People 2010*. Rockville, MD: Office of Disease Prevention and Health Promotion. www.healthypeople.gov/2010/Publications/.

Weinreich, N. K. 1999. *Hands-On Social Marketing: A Step-by-Step Guide*. Thousand Oaks, CA: Sage Publications.

World Health Organization (WHO). 2013. "World Health Statistics: Life Expectancy at Birth, Both Sexes, 2011." http://gamapserver.who.int/gho/interactive_charts/mbd/life_expectancy /atlas.html.

———. 2010. "Global Vaccine Safety: Q&A on Myths and Facts About Vaccination Available." www.who.int/immunization_safety/aefi/immunization_misconceptions/en/.

CHAPTER 9

THE PRESENCE OF POLITICS

LEARNING OBJECTIVES

After studying this chapter, you will be able to

➤ explain the concept of the presence of politics in healthcare;

➤ examine the impact of politics and power by virtue of position on healthcare marketing endeavors;

➤ recognize the impact of politics on healthcare employees;

➤ describe the function of patients, physicians, payers, and the public in healthcare marketing initiatives; and

➤ evaluate the role of the healthcare marketer in relation to the presence of politics.

CASE STUDY: REMEMBERING CARIBOU CLINICS

Stephen Bergman (director of Caribou Medical Clinics Foundation), Nancy Colbert (director of marketing and communications), and Robin Hughes (director of news and internal relations) took a break from their work to eat lunch in the Caribou Foundation conference room. All morning they had been working on their latest team project, *Remembering Caribou,* and they had decided to keep at it for the rest of the day. Stephen took a moment to acknowledge the good work they had accomplished so far. "You know, this is a project to be proud of. We have developed a planned giving program that will encourage stakeholders to establish annuities for Caribou and remember Caribou in their wills. Our goal is to obtain 175 of these legacy gifts within the next year, and I think we are on the right track."

Nancy nodded her head in agreement, took a sip of her bottled water, and said, "I like this partnership. We have been able to strategize our plan, and eventually I think we will have a turnkey program that will be easily applied throughout our regions. Robin, have we forgotten any outlets for communications?"

Robin looked down at her iPad to read her notes regarding **distribution avenues** and materials:

distribution avenues channels through which information, a product, or a service is communicated or made available to target markets

Title of Project	Remembering Caribou
Distribution avenues	1. *Direct mailing* to donors and prospective donors
	2. *Regional television:* appearances on various local talk shows; commercials showcasing stories of patients who are willing to share their Caribou experiences
	3. *Radio:* appearances on various local radio talk shows; commercials showcasing stories of patients who are willing to share their Caribou experiences
	4. *Newspaper:* articles that highlight the *Remembering Caribou* program
	5. *Annual 5k run/walk:* highlight *Remembering Caribou* message during this annual fundraiser
	6. *One-on-one conversations:* board members' initiative
Materials	1. Brochures
	2. Flyers
	3. DVD and USB flash drives
	4. Internal newsletter to Caribou employees
	5. External newsletter to public, physicians, and patients

Robin looked up from her iPad and said, "We don't have billboards listed. Do we want to add them?"

Stephen and Nancy exchanged looks. Stephen spoke first. "Dr. Metzger will want to use billboards. Nancy, you worked with him on the marketing campaign about our purchase of the da Vinci robot five years ago for the Heart Institute, remember?"

Nancy remembered it—almost too well. The da Vinci robot marketing campaign had been given a budget of $80,000 to communicate the acquisition of the first robotic surgery platform in the region, and Dr. Metzger had insisted that 75 percent of it—$60,000—be spent on billboards. At first, Nancy had resisted Dr. Metzger's desire to have his and his colleagues' pictures plastered on billboards around the city. In her opinion, it was vain at best, and the use of billboards would limit their ability to reach the targeted market; it would have communicated the da Vinci robot purchase only to automobile drivers in one city.

One afternoon, the CEO of the hospital summoned Nancy to her office to discuss the project. During their meeting, the CEO explained that she had spoken with Dr. Metzger and that he was adamant that the billboards be included in the marketing campaign. In fact, Dr. Metzger wanted the entire budget spent on billboards so that he and his colleagues could be featured in other cities, too.

In the end, the CEO granted Dr. Metzger his wish, and the billboards made up practically the entire communications campaign and consumed most of the budget. Nancy was never able to determine how much of the cardiovascular market they had reached, given that other communication avenues had been eliminated. Of course, Dr. Metzger was pleased with the campaign.

Interrupting Nancy's thoughts, Stephen continued, "And, we do not want to exclude any of our market (donors and potential donors) because we did not consider their requests. Billboards will take up a chunk of our budget, but Dr. Metzger is on the foundation board." He pointed to Robin's iPad and said, "Add billboards. We don't need the 'elephant' to roll over us."

Robin looked confused. Nancy laughed and tried to help her understand. "Robin, what do you do if you are in bed with an elephant?"

Robin still looked confused, and Stephen chimed in, "Anything to make certain that the elephant doesn't roll over you!"

Robin thought her colleagues' humor was weird, but then she got it. "Oh! The elephant is Dr. Metzger. Okay! Billboards it is!"

HEALTHCARE MARKETING AND POLITICS

In Chapter 5, *politics* was defined as "social relations involving authority or power" (die. net) as well as "a strife of interests masquerading as a contest of principles; the conduct of public affairs for private advantage" (Bierce 1993, 95). As the case study demonstrates, politics—specifically organizational politics—is present in activities throughout healthcare, even in marketing campaigns like *Remembering Caribou*. In a classic article on the subject published in 1977, **organizational politics** is defined as "the management of influence to obtain ends not sanctioned by the organization or to obtain sanctioned ends through non-sanctioned influence means" (Mayes and Allen 1977, 675). The article presented the table in Exhibit 9.1 to illustrate how this definition applies in an organization.

In the context of healthcare organizations, each quadrant in Exhibit 9.1 represents different kinds of healthcare activities. Quadrant I is nonpolitical job behavior. For example, the meeting between Nancy, Stephen, and Robin fits in this quadrant. They are putting together a plan for the *Remembering Caribou* campaign while being mindful of budget, process, and outcomes. They are simply doing their jobs.

Quadrant II represents political behaviors that comprise both sanctioned and non-sanctioned actions. For example, consider events that might occur after research has identified a clinical process that benefits patients, such as frequent hand washing (Backman, Zoutman, and Marck 2008; Pirie 2010). Since professional acceptance of the importance of hand washing for reducing infection became widespread, marketing campaigns have encouraged all hospital staff to wash their hands between each contact they have with patients. Tip #10 included in AHRQ's 2011 publication *20 Tips to Help Prevent Medical Errors* reminds patients not to allow healthcare workers to touch them unless they have washed their hands (see www.ahrq.gov/consumer/20tips.htm). Marketing materials on hand washing for healthcare professionals, such as the hand hygiene poster provided by the Massachusetts Department of Health (see www.mass.gov/eohhs/docs/dph/cdc/handwashing/hand-hygiene-poster.pdf), are often available free of charge.

Given that research has identified the benefits of hand washing and that the government and hospital protocol support hand washing, one would expect healthcare workers to comply—yet some do not. This refusal to comply is represented by Quadrant II. For instance, say a physician who has been granted admitting privileges by a hospital refuses to

organizational politics behavior aimed at self-gain, regardless of whether it brings about gain for others

Influence Means	Influence Ends	
	Organizationally Sanctioned	*Not Sanctioned by Organization*
Organizationally sanctioned	Nonpolitical job behavior (Quadrant I)	Organizationally dysfunctional political behavior (Quadrant II)
Not sanctioned by organization	Political behavior potentially functional to the organization (Quadrant III)	Organizationally dysfunctional political behavior (Quadrant IV)

EXHIBIT 9.1
Dimensions of Organizational Politics

Source: Mayes and Allen (1977, 675).

do so because he thinks it takes too much time and knows that nobody can make him comply. The hospital has sanctioned the physician's practice of admitting and treating patients in the hospital, but the physician's refusal to follow recommended hand-washing procedures is organizationally dysfunctional behavior that has the potential to increase the rate of infection among his patients. (In one study, researchers reviewed assessments of healthcare providers' compliance with hand-washing recommendations and found that approximately 32 percent of physicians practiced good hand hygiene [Erasmus et al. 2010].)

Quadrant III refers to actions that are not officially sanctioned by an organization but support its function and contribute to its outcomes. One example illustrative of Quadrant III behavior concerns patients with cancer during the 1970s. At that time, patients had fewer options for transportation to hospitals for chemotherapy sessions than they do today. They could have someone drive them, take a taxi, or take public transportation. Volunteer programs that provide rides to chemotherapy sessions, such as that offered by the American Cancer Society, were not organized as efficiently as they are today. A women's organization on a college campus learned about a young lady who was missing chemotherapy treatments because she could not find transportation to the hospital. The organization put together a volunteer driving program (albeit short lived) to transport local patients to their treatment facilities. The hospitals did not formally sanction this service, but the service supported and helped them provide patient care.

Quadrant IV refers to organizationally dysfunctional political behavior that is not sanctioned by an organization. Because such actions are not tolerated, anyone engaged in such behavior does so secretively. For this reason, assessment of Quadrant IV behavior is "resistant to research attempts" (Mayes and Allen 1977, 676).

POLITICS AND POSITION POWER

With reference to the case study and the dimensions of organizational politics presented in Exhibit 9.1, the da Vinci robot campaign and the billboard situation fit in Quadrant II. Dr. Metzger has privileges and is sanctioned by the hospital to provide patient care. He also is a member of the foundation board. Yet his behavior during the da Vinci robot marketing campaign was organizationally dysfunctional because his self-interest in appearing larger than life on billboards compromised the campaign's aim of reaching all targeted markets.

A prominent article published in 1989 added a component to organizational politics, defining it as a "behavior [that] is strategically designed to maximize short-term or long-term self-interest, which is either consistent with or at the expense of others' interests" (Ferris, Russ, and Fandt 1989, 145). In other words, political behavior might or might not support others' interests in addition to one's own. This definition and Quadrant II of the model in Exhibit 9.1 both apply to Dr. Metzger's stance regarding the billboards.

However, although Dr. Metzger made his stance known, he did not actually execute it. The mere thought that Dr. Metzger might react as he did before encouraged the *Remembering Caribou* team to include billboards in their campaign plan. This indirect influence is called **power**. Dr. Metzger possesses **power by virtue of position**. A study of the relationship between organizational politics and power conducted in 1980 concluded that organizational politics and power are interrelated (Madison et al. 1980, 97):

> [I]t is not the direct exercise of authority *per se* that is perceived as political. . . . [P]erceived political activity is an influence attempt outside the traditional use of authority to direct the activity of others.

The billboard campaign is outside the traditional domain of Dr. Metzger's **authority** as a physician. Nonetheless, as discussed in Chapter 5, many physicians refer patients to hospitals but are not employed by those hospitals. At the same time, physicians are dependent on hospitals to provide healthcare facilities for medical practice. The relationship is mutually interdependent: Physicians need hospitals, and hospitals need physicians. Given this political relationship, marketing efforts such as *Remembering Caribou* are highly likely to incorporate physicians' wishes.

However, as the number of physicians moving away from private practice toward hospital- or corporate-based employment increases, this relationship may change. The Medical Group Management Association reports that about 65 percent of established physicians and 49 percent of physicians hired out of school were employees of hospital-owned practices in 2009 (MGMA 2010). Organizations' responses to physician employees engaged in organizational politics may differ from their responses to referring physicians in private practice; while hospitals and physicians will remain interdependent, physicians' base of power will change.

ORGANIZATIONAL POLITICS AND THE WORKPLACE

More recent research regarding organizational politics focuses on perceptions of organizational politics and the effect, if any, the perception of the presence (or absence) of politics has on work stress, job satisfaction, job turnover, and organizational commitment (i.e., loyalty) of staff members (Chang, Rosen, and Levy 2009; Miller, Rutherford, and Kokodinsky 2008). A review of more than 50 studies addressing these effects revealed that workers who perceived the presence of organizational politics had lower job satisfaction and were less committed to their organization than were those who did not have this perception. Moreover, workers with this perception reported greater job stress and turnover intentions (Miller, Rutherford, and Kokodinsky 2008).

power
the ability to influence someone else to take some action, regardless of whether he or she wants to do so

power by virtue of position
the ability to influence someone else to take some action, regardless of whether he or she wants to do so, derived from the authority awarded to the influencer's position

authority
the ability of someone in a position of power to direct others to take some action

HEALTHCARE MARKETERS AS CRITICAL THINKERS AND CREATIVE PROBLEM SOLVERS

It is important for healthcare marketers to recognize and fully comprehend organizational politics. It might be frustrating and stressful to design a marketing plan that is consistent with an organization's mission and financially sound only to have it changed significantly via organizational politics and the influence of power. To respond as best as possible to the presence of politics, one should be mindful of the organization's mission and work in an ethical manner. Because it is stressful to deal with politics and the people who play politics, this task is easier said than done.

The Mission

Any healthcare marketing initiative (e.g., *Remembering Caribou*) should fit well with the mission of an organization. At the same time, those involved in the planning and implementation of healthcare marketing projects should be mindful of the organization's stakeholders—the people and groups that have a stake in the enterprise and are affected by the conduct of people within it. Their behavior should follow the ethical standards discussed in Chapter 4:

- *Justice:* This standard emphasizes the importance of proper and appropriate behavior and equal treatment among patients, physicians, payers, and the public.

- *Fidelity:* This standard concerns loyalty; faithfulness to duty; and respect for patients, physicians, payers, and the public. Healthcare marketers are loyal to their workplace as well as mindful of the environment and community in which they live.

- *Beneficence:* This standard refers to the professional duty to benefit others.

- *Autonomy:* This standard is based on the premise that people are able to make informed decisions that respect and consider the well-being of patients, physicians, payers, and the public.

Consider the mission statements of St. Jude Children's Research Hospital, Greene County Health Care, Intermountain Healthcare, Eastern Idaho Regional Medical Center, and Caribou Clinics (the site in the case study):

St. Jude Children's Research Hospital (2013) conducts pediatric research and provides healthcare at no charge to its patients:

The mission of St. Jude Children's Research Hospital is to advance cures, and means of prevention, for pediatric catastrophic diseases through research and treatment. Consistent with the vision of our founder Danny Thomas, no child is denied treatment based on race, religion or a family's ability to pay.

Greene County Health Care (2011) provides healthcare to persons who earn 200 percent of the federal poverty level or less; 87 percent of its patients are uninsured:

The mission of Greene County Health Care is to ensure the availability of quality health care to all residents of Greene, Pitt and Pamlico Counties and the surrounding rural area with an emphasis on providing health services to the underserved.

Intermountain Healthcare (2013) provides healthcare for patients in Utah and southeastern Idaho:

Excellence in the provision of healthcare services to communities in the Intermountain region.

Eastern Idaho Regional Medical Center (2009) provides healthcare to persons in Idaho and surrounding regions; its corporate parent is HCA:

To improve the lives of those we touch.

Caribou Clinics is the site in this chapter's case study:

As people of Caribou, we strive to provide exceptional and innovative care to patients, families, and the community through delivery of the finest clinical care while respecting the needs of the human spirit.

The missions of these five healthcare organizations have common ground. All are focused on delivering healthcare to their "people," whether the people are children at St. Jude or persons in Greene County, North Carolina. So, while politics may exist and may influence the implementation of marketing plans, it is important to focus on how the marketing endeavor ties into and reinforces the mission of the organization. This focus reinforces the purpose of the work professionals in healthcare marketing do (or aspire to do).

Consider the characters in the case study at the beginning of this chapter, and identify their course of action. What factors should they keep in mind as they plan the campaign? How do the standards of justice, fidelity, beneficence, and autonomy guide them? For the planning team of Stephen, Nancy, and Robin, the ultimate goal is the success of

Remembering Caribou and the funds the campaign will raise. These funds will help Caribou carry out its mission.

The team members are aware that politics is present in healthcare, so they were quick to include billboards as a method of communication. The use of billboards may not be the most cost-effective means of delivering the campaign's message, but Stephen, Nancy, and Robin acknowledge the adage about "being in bed with the elephant." The elephant has power, and their proactive inclusion of the billboards stays the course of Caribou Clinics' mission (and ensures that the elephant does not roll over them).

By understanding and evaluating others' behavior in terms of politics, one can better predict what they might do and then engage in actions that will yield benefits and advantages for oneself and others (Robbins 2003, 162). By pleasing Dr. Metzger, the team might be able to turn him into one of the 175 who "remember Caribou" through a legacy gift—the goal of the campaign.

CHAPTER QUESTIONS

1. As noted in this chapter, physicians are moving away from private practice toward hospital- and corporate-based employment. Consider Dr. Metzger and his desire for the billboard campaign. If he were a salaried employee instead of a referring physician in private practice, would the marketers include the billboards as part of their plan? Create a scenario in which they include the billboards, and explain why they decided to do so. Then create a scenario in which they do not include the billboards, and explain why they made this decision.

2. Think of an example in your community where communications from a healthcare facility probably had been influenced by the presence of politics. For example, have you seen billboards picturing physicians who practice in your town?

3. Go to St. Jude's website (www.stjude.org), and examine its marketing communications about its fundraising initiatives. How do these communications fit with St. Jude's mission?

CHAPTER EXERCISES

1. *What if it were a nurse?*

   In the case study at the beginning of this chapter, the subject matter centered on the team members' response to the physician. Reread the case study but substitute a nurse for Dr. Metzger. If a nurse had wanted what the physician wanted, what do you think the response would have been? Why? Relate your response to the concept of power by virtue of position.

2. *St. Jude's mission and marketing efforts*

    Describe three marketing projects that tie into St. Jude's mission, and explain why they fit. (Hint: Go to St. Jude's website for ideas [www.stjude.org/waystohelp].)

REFERENCES

Agency for Healthcare Research and Quality (AHRQ). 2011. *20 Tips to Help Prevent Medical Errors*. AHRQ Publication # 11-0089. Current as of September. www.ahrq.gov/consumer/20tips.htm.

Backman, D., D. Zoutman, and P. Marck. 2008. "An Integrative Review of the Current Evidence on the Relationship Between Hand Hygiene Interventions and the Incidence of Health Care–Associated Infections." *American Journal of Infection Control* 36 (5): 333–48.

Bierce, A. 1993. *The Devil's Dictionary*. Mineola, NY: Dover Publications, Inc.

Chang, C. H., C. C. Rosen, and P. E. Levy. 2009. "The Relationship Between Perceptions of Organizational Politics and Employee Attitudes, Strain, and Behavior: A Meta-Analytic Examination." *Academy of Management Journal* 52 (4): 779–801.

Eastern Idaho Regional Medical Center. 2009. "About Our Hospital." http://eirmc.com/about/.

Erasmus, V., T. Daha, H. Brug, J. Richardus, M. Behrendt, M. Vos, and E. Beeck. 2010. "Systematic Review of Studies on Compliance with Hand Hygiene Guidelines in Hospital Care." *Infection Control and Hospital Epidemiology* 31 (3): 283–94.

Ferris, G., G. Russ, and P. Fandt. 1989. "Politics in Organizations." In *Impression Management in the Organization*, edited by R. Giacalone and P. Rosenfeld, 143–70. Hillsdale, NJ: Lawrence Erlbaum.

Greene County Health Care. 2011. Home page. www.greenecountyhealthcare.com/.

Intermountain Healthcare. 2013. "Mission, Vision, Values." http://intermountainhealth care.org/about/overview/Pages/mission.aspx.

Madison, D., R. Allen, L. Porter, P. Renwick, and B. Mayes. 1980. "Organizational Politics: An Exploration of Managers' Perceptions." *Human Relations* 33 (2): 79–100.

Mayes, B., and R. Allen. 1977. "Toward a Definition of Organizational Politics." *Academy of Management Review* 2 (4): 672–78.

Medical Group Management Association (MGMA). 2010. "MGMA Physician Placement Report: 65 Percent of Established Physicians Placed in Hospital-Owned Practices." Press release, June 3. www.mgma.com/press/default.aspx?id=33777.

Miller, B., M. Rutherford, and R. Kokodinsky. 2008. "Perceptions of Organizational Politics: A Meta-Analysis of Outcomes." *Journal of Business and Psychology* 22: 209–22.

Pirie, S. 2010. "Hand Washing and Surgical Hand Antisepsis." *Journal of Perioperative Practice* 20 (5): 169–72.

Robbins, S. 2003. *Essentials of Organizational Behavior*, seventh edition. Upper Saddle River, NJ: Prentice Hall.

St. Jude Children's Research Hospital. 2013. "St. Jude Mission Statement." www.stjude.org /stjude/v/index.jsp?vgnextoid=9dc4b8ca05604210VgnVCM1000001e0215acRCRD&vgn extchannel=f67c1e3d40419210VgnVCM1000001e0215acRCRD.

PART III

INTERPERSONAL SKILLS FOR THE HEALTHCARE MARKETER

This real-life case introduces students to common healthcare marketplace issues and controversies related to specialty hospitals and hospital–physician joint ventures. It also exposes students to examples of interpersonal and interprofessional conflict, inadequate and poorly aligned organizational communication strategies, and inept leadership and teamwork that often lead— as in this case—to poor organizational performance. Participant and facility names and various numerical values have been modified to preserve anonymity and accentuate points of learning.

This case challenges students to consider organizational and marketplace realities when pursuing strategic initiatives, including the need for proactive insurance/managed care contracting, sound financial and business modeling, and credible marketing strategies and plans. The material presented in Part III of this text focuses on helping students effectively manage conflict, improve their leadership skills and teamwork, communicate the right messages to the community, and address other important strategic marketing questions.

SPECIALTY HOSPITAL PROS AND CONS

Advocates argue that specialty hospitals provide higher-quality care at lower per unit costs by concentrating physician skills and other hospital/medical resources on managing complex diseases (Nallamothu et al. 2007). Critics contend that specialty hospitals focus largely on low-risk patients and shift the financial burden of uncompensated care to competing general hospitals. Opponents further argue that physician ownership of specialty hospitals incentivizes physicians to refer patients to their own facilities, cherry-pick low-risk and well-insured patients, and induce demand for certain services (Al-Amin et al. 2010).

but cost shifting is acceptable? or not?

RATIONALE FOR HOSPITAL–PHYSICIAN JOINT VENTURES

The overarching goal of a hospital–physician joint venture is to create a clinical and economic entity that benefits patients and the physicians and hospital(s) participating in it. Patient/community benefits include improved processes of care, services, and outcomes. Potential benefits for participating physicians include opportunities for increased revenues, more efficient use of time, and greater control over operational matters affecting patient care and physician convenience. Benefits for the participating hospital include the maintenance of profitable revenue streams if physician investors sign covenants not to invest in competing facilities (Cohn et al. 2005).

PALOMAR HEART HOSPITAL

Palomar Heart Hospital (PHH), a provider of cardiology-related services to patients living in and around the Central Valley of California, opened its doors in 2003. The opening of this $50 million state-of-the-art facility was consistent with the nationwide proliferation of physician-owned and hospital–physician joint-ventured specialty hospitals in the early 2000s (Barro, Huckman, and Kessler 2006). PHH was a 51/49 joint venture between Lincoln Healthcare System (LHS) and Central Valley area cardiologists and cardiothoracic surgeons, respectively.

Russell Taylor joined LHS as executive vice president/chief operating officer (EVP/COO) the same month PHH opened its doors. Russell was the third EVP/COO hired in the past 24 months to lead a systemwide financial turnaround of the ailing vertically and horizontally integrated four-hospital healthcare system.

Notwithstanding the PHH facility's physical attractiveness and first-rate technology, PHH lost between $700,000 and $1.1 million per month during its first six months of operation. Expected monthly losses/gains during this period ranged from –$150,000 to $250,000. Losses at PHH not only far exceeded LHS's worst expectations but also contributed significantly to the continued overall underperformance of LHS. After corporate management's repeated but unsuccessful attempts to persuade Phil Surrowitz, PHH's founding CEO, to adjust and improve PHH's marketing and staffing plans and better manage overall expenses, the decision was made to replace him. Although Russell's span of control stretched across LHS, he knew that stopping the financial hemorrhage at PHH was his first and highest priority. In consultation with other LHS executives, physicians, and trusted staff, Russell identified the central issues leading to PHH's woeful financial and operating performance:

◆   PHH's leaders were ineffective and neither willing nor able to make the difficult decisions needed to improve the hospital's marketing and operations.

◆   Conflict existed among area cardiologists and cardiothoracic surgeons. From the outset, jealousies and hard feelings among several of the seven founding physicians/surgeons (each of whom had a substantive ownership interest in PHH) led certain cardiologists to refuse to refer patients to their fellow PHH heart surgeons and vice versa.

◆   Teamwork among key PHH and LHS personnel was poor. Notwithstanding its 49 percent physician ownership, PHH was an important member of the LHS family of hospitals and related healthcare facilities. Yet PHH's managers resisted assistance and oversight from LHS's corporate personnel, including finance/accounting, marketing/planning, and insurance contracting specialists who were able and willing to assist.

◆   PHH had insufficient and inappropriate contracts with health insurance plans. Although PHH's managers had been given more than two years' advance notice to negotiate managed care/insurance contracts to ensure adequate patient volumes, roughly 40 percent of the area population was unable to use PHH's services because their HMO or commercial insurance plan had not yet negotiated terms with PHH.

◆   PHH's cost structure was suffocating. Because of its first-rate construction, technology, costly furnishings, rich staffing mix, and highly paid staff, the hospital needed to perform 45 invasive surgeries/procedures and 280 outpatient procedures per month and maintain an average daily census of 30 patients just to break even financially. In light of competing hospital-based cardiology programs and long-standing strained relations among PHH physicians and surgeons, Russell wondered if other services, including general, bariatric, and colorectal surgery; endoscopy; and other medical/surgical services should be added to PHH's repertoire to increase patient volume and revenues and offset overhead expenses. The idea of adding non-cardiology services to this premier regional heart hospital was not well received by the cardiologist and cardiac surgeon owners. Board members, employees, and other LHS managers questioned the wisdom of adjusting the facility's mission and core scope of services so soon after opening, while a growing chorus of dissenters argued otherwise.

◆ PHH had ineffective marketing plans. Phil Surrowitz enjoyed "good old boy" standing among many of the area's cardiologists, so he did not consider using traditional marketing methods to attract the attention and ultimate business of insurers, primary care physicians, and patients.

◆ PHH's key managers, physicians, and surgeons had poor financial literacy. Although the CEO and senior financial officer understood the hospital's financial picture, few other managers and employees—including the physician owners—fully appreciated the financial dynamics and nuances.

A summary of select projected and actual financial and operating indicators from PHH's first six months of operation is provided in Exhibit 1.

NEXT STEPS

Russell knew he needed to provide an overview of PHH's performance to date and a compelling plan for improvement at the upcoming meeting of the LHS board. Because various board members still questioned LHS's specialty hospital strategy and the purpose of the PHH joint venture, an overview of the pros and cons of specialty hospitals and hospital–physician joint ventures in general was also in order.

DISCUSSION QUESTIONS

1. What are some of the apparent advantages and disadvantages of specialty hospitals from a patient/family perspective? From a physician/hospital perspective? From a community perspective?
2. What are some advantages of participating in hospital–physician joint ventures in terms of a hospital's or health system's overall strategy?
3. What planning and marketing techniques could Russell and his team use to improve the financial and operating performance of PHH?
4. In your judgment, is it too soon to amend the mission, vision, and/or scope of services offered by PHH? Why or why not?
5. What sources of conflict contributed to PHH's poor performance? What leadership and teamwork strategies would you employ to address these conflicts and improve performance?
6. What steps could Russell take to address the interpersonal conflicts with PHH?

Exhibit 1
Palomar Heart Hospital: Select Operating and Financial* Data

	Jan		Feb		Mar		Apr		May		Jun		YTD	
	Actual	Projected	Actual	Projected	Actual	Projected	Actual	Projected	Actual	Projected	Actual	Projected	Actual	Projected
Average daily census[1]	12	24	14	28	15	28	16	30	17	30	17	32	15.2	28.6
Invasive surgeries/procedures[2]	18	30	19	35	19	40	22	45	32	50	31	55	141	255
Outpatient procedures[3]	130	225	139	240	119	265	137	280	167	305	169	330	861	1,645
Medicare percentage (discharges)	66	65	67	65	63	65	65	65	69	65	67	65	66	65
Net revenues[4]	$750	$1,810	$960	$1,991	$1,066	$2,091	$1,242	$2,195	$1,592	$2,327	$1,798	$2,475	$7,408	$12,889
Total expenses[5]	$1,850	$1,960	$2,010	$2,091	$2,016	$2,141	$2,117	$2,195	$2,442	$2,202	$2,523	$2,225	$12,958	$12,814
Net operating income[6]	($1,100)	($150)	($1,050)	($100)	($950)	($50)	($875)	$0	($850)	$125	($725)	$250	($5,550)	$75
Days cash on hand (LHS)[7]	93	95	90	96	86	97	82	98	78	99	75	100	75	100

*In thousands of dollars.

1. Average daily census (ADC) is a measure of inpatient volume. It is a function of both discharges and length of stay. In today's fixed payment systems, increases in ADC ideally should come from increases in discharges rather than from increases in length of stay.
2. Invasive surgeries/procedures include coronary artery bypass surgery, angioplasty, atherectomy, cardiomyoplasty, radiofrequency oblation, stent procedures, and more.
3. Outpatient procedures include treadmill testing, electrocardiography, 24-hour holter monitoring, nuclear cardiology, pacemaker and defibrillator checkups, and more.
4. Net revenues are approximately 37 percent of gross revenues.
5. Total expenses are the sum of all labor and nonlabor expenses, including corporate overhead.
6. Net operating income includes total net revenues less total expenses.
7. Days cash on hand (LHS) measures the number of days LHS could pay for its average daily expenses with the cash and marketable securities it has. It is an important measure of total liquidity.

REFERENCES

Al-Amin, M., J. Zinn, M. Rosko, and W. Aaronson. 2010. "Specialty Hospital Market Proliferation: Strategic Imperatives for General Hospitals." *Health Care Management Review* 35 (4): 294–300.

Barro, J. R., R. S. Huckman, and D. P. Kessler. 2006. "The Effects of Cardiac Specialty Hospitals on the Cost and Quality of Medical Care." *Journal of Health Economics* 25 (4): 702–21.

Cohn, K. H., T. R. Allyn, R. H. Y. Rosenfield, and R. Schwartz. 2005. "Overview of Physician–Hospital Ventures." *American Journal of Surgery* 189 (1): 4–10.

Nallamothu, B. K., M. A. Rogers, M. E. Chernew, H. M. Krumholz, K. Eagle, and J. D. Birkmeyer. 2007. "Opening of Specialty Cardiac Hospitals and Use of Coronary Revascularization in Medicare Beneficiaries." *Journal of the American Medical Association* 297 (9): 962–68.

CHAPTER 10

COMMUNICATION

LEARNING OBJECTIVES

After studying this chapter, you will be able to

➤ identify the special circumstances inherent in health marketing communications,

➤ persuasively argue for the importance of consistency of message and alignment in health marketing communications,

➤ distinguish between internal and external health marketing communications, and

➤ define relationship marketing.

CASE STUDY: BRINGING HEALTHCARE MARKETING INTO THE TWENTY-FIRST CENTURY

Kenji Katsuya had been doing freelance marketing for a number of small health organizations in rural Utah for five years and had earned a reputation for excellence and professionalism. His marketing communications were visually appealing, clear, consistent, and informative. He and his wife were expecting their first child, and they decided that he should seek a position in an organization instead of continuing his freelance work. One of his clients told him that a small critical access hospital in the area, Ute River Hospital, was looking for a new head of marketing. He applied for the position and got it.

During his interview at Ute River, Kenji learned that the outgoing head of marketing had retired about two years earlier after having worked there for more than 30 years. At first, Ute River's CEO had thought that she didn't need to replace him. After all, Ute River was the only hospital within a 75-mile radius; it had no real competition other than the large hospitals in the Salt Lake City area. Instead of maintaining a separate marketing department, the hospital allotted each of its departments an equal amount from the marketing budget to produce its own marketing materials. After two years, the CEO changed her mind and decided to hire a marketing head.

Even after learning that the hospital had not had a marketing department or head for two years, Kenji was surprised and a bit shocked when he saw Ute River's marketing communications. Some departments had constructed homemade flyers with copier paper of various colors. On many of the pieces they had used multiple fonts, underlining, and boldface. The text contained misspellings and incorrect grammar, and the messages were confusing. Other departments had large signs featuring photos of Ute River's patients and caregivers. Some had created their own logos. Others had no communications at all. The marketing materials the previous marketing head had developed for the hospital itself were outdated. Ute River wasn't running print, radio, television, or electronic advertisements and didn't even have a website.

But the crazy quilt of marketing materials wasn't Kenji's only problem. The department heads were angry about having to return their marketing funds to re-create a central marketing budget. Many expressed hostility toward him outright, particularly when they found out that the new marketing budget was nearly triple what it had been under the old marketing head.

Kenji knew, however, that he had the strong support of the CEO and the board. The increase in the marketing budget was a clear message that the organization was ready to move its marketing communications forward. Kenji's job was to create a consistent, professional image of Ute River Hospital and find the best marketing media and channels for it. He was ready for the challenge.

COMMUNICATING IN HEALTHCARE

Everyone is familiar with the basic idea of communication. One person, the sender, wants to convey information to another person, the receiver. The sender conveys the information over a **communication channel**, perhaps by speaking or writing, and the receiver hears or reads it and interprets it. The true goal of communication is for the sender to transmit the information so clearly and perfectly and for the receiver to hear it so precisely that the receiver understands it exactly as the sender intended it to be understood. On the surface, this concept seems fundamental and simple, but myriad factors can obstruct communication, including language, nonverbal cues, emotions, and background noise, to name just a few.

communication channel
the method or medium through which a message or information is communicated

In healthcare marketing, communication can be especially difficult because the message one is trying to send is often complex and needs to be fine-tuned to specific audiences. Healthcare is a highly emotional, personal subject; for this reason, health communications need to be sensitive, nonjudgmental, and inoffensive. Traditionally, marketing communication has been thought of in terms of advertising and promotion. While both are of great importance in healthcare marketing, health communication often concerns far more than sales; for example, it may focus on public health, social marketing, or health education. Health marketing communication might seem to be all about the sender and the message being sent, but it is not. Despite the importance of the sender and the message, excellent health marketing communication is perhaps even more about the receiver and what that person hears and understands. Therefore, healthcare marketers need to listen to their audience or target market to ensure it will understand and accept the messages they send.

LISTENING

Everyone has had the experience of speaking before an audience that isn't paying attention or listening. And all have had someone "talk at" them when they are not interested in hearing what that person has to say. Amid the cacophony of marketing and advertising in the world, what does the consumer actually hear? How do healthcare marketers ensure that their audiences pay attention to the communications they create and send, absorb the messages above the fray, and accurately interpret what they are hearing?

Listeners are highly diverse with regard to education, ethnicity, age, language, health condition, and their understanding of health and wellness. According to census information from 2011, "for the first time, racial and ethnic minorities make up more than half the children born in the US" (Yen 2012). In addition, the US population comprises four distinct adult generations—the Silent Generation (those born between 1900 and 1945), the Baby Boomers (1946–1964), Generation X (1965–1980), and "Millennials" or Generation Y (1981–present)—each having its own needs, issues, and communication channels and styles. Listeners are becoming increasingly savvy and skeptical about advertising and promotion, and they have short attention spans, particularly when the communication misses the mark.

Listeners absorb and understand messages more fully when little background noise is present and the message is of interest to them. Healthcare marketers need to meet their listeners where they are and align their message to that time and place. Too many health marketing messages are based on what the marketer assumes about the listener, what the marketer thinks the listener needs to hear, or even worse, what the marketer herself would like to hear. **Message alignment** is a complex concept. How does a person's cultural background, for example, influence her health and wellness behavior and her use (or nonuse) of health services? Why does someone choose one physician, hospital, or clinic over another? To answer such questions, one must have an in-depth knowledge of the market, the target audience, and the competition. Healthcare marketers need to conduct excellent marketing research, of course, but they also need to be good listeners themselves.

message alignment
the synchronization and consistency of a message with the receiver's culture, knowledge, and interests

COMMUNICATION CHANNELS

Marketing communication is both a science and an art. The science is the knowledge and skills needed to manipulate, draft, and send messages and information to the desired receivers. The art is the creation of effective, timely, and sensitive communication that touches the listener and influences him to respond in a specific way. In the not-so-distant past, newspapers, mail, radio, television, and live events were the primary channels for all marketing. Today, an almost limitless number of communication channels are available to healthcare marketers: websites, social media, blogs, e-mail, health records, newspapers, "robo calls," radio, television, snail mail, billboards, flyers, pop-up advertisements, and so forth. Successful healthcare marketing orchestrates an optimal mix of communication channels and messages. Allowing individual departments or professionals to create their own marketing materials and messages can spell disaster. While the actual channels used may vary, one thing is certain: The overarching message needs to be consistent; align with the organization's mission, vision, and goals; and have an identifiable look and feel. Marketers must work with all personnel in the organization to ensure they create an accurate, timely, unified message. Marketing communications are the vehicle of an organization's **brand management**.

brand management
controlling and influencing the relationship between an organization's customers and its readily identifiable and publicly recognized products or services

Consistency can begin with elements as simple as color, font, logo, and tagline and can be as complex as tacit imagery. For example, what do people associate with a picture of a man and a woman in separate bathtubs overlooking a scenic view? Many immediately think of a medication for erectile dysfunction. The line "because I'm worth it" brings women's hair coloring and makeup to mind. Bathtubs and "being worth it" are excellent examples of highly effective, consistent images/slogans that immediately identify and brand a product.

Even though health organizations and caregivers provide incredibly diverse and highly personalized products, nearly all of them use the terms *high-quality care* or *personalized care* in their mission statements and marketing messages (Bolon 2005). Nothing is wrong with these terms, but because nearly every health provider uses them, they do not differentiate one provider from another and are thus unmemorable.

EVERYONE IS A MARKETER

In the past, marketing was done by marketing departments. They produced print and oral communications geared toward a target audience or the public. Other healthcare workers, in particular caregivers, never thought of themselves as marketers. However, in today's competitive healthcare environment, leaving marketing solely to the marketing department is sorely inadequate. Everyone from the board president and CEO to caregivers, technicians, and custodians needs to see himself as part of the marketing team. When a physician or nurse is brusque with a patient or colleague, she sends the patient a message about the care the organization provides. When a patient is kept on hold but repeatedly told by an automated voice that her "call is important to us," the organization sends a clear message that the call is not important. When facility direction signs and health education materials are not translated into Spanish, particularly in cities with large Hispanic and Latino populations, a message is communicated. When physicians are always referred to as "he" and with the title "doctor" and nurses are always referred to as "she" and by their first names, it sends a message. Regardless of how on-point and perfectly targeted the marketing department's external communications are, day-to-day internal communications, actions, and experiences such as those just described create dissonance.

Every time someone with the organization has contact with a patient or consumer, regardless if it is in person, by word of mouth, written, electronic, or visual, he is sending a marketing/branding communication that speaks loudly about the organization. Sometimes these contacts are called **brand touch points** or **brand contact points**.

RELATIONSHIP, RELATIONSHIP, RELATIONSHIP

The old way of thinking held that marketing was about advertising and selling. This idea is outdated, particularly in healthcare, where the lines between buyers, sellers, customers, and payers are blurred. Today's healthcare marketing is about building and maintaining relationships between patients, providers, and health organizations; between health organizations and payers; and between volunteers, donors, and health facilities. All relationships are built on mutual need, service, and trust. According to a 2012 Gallup poll, the top three of the five most honest and ethical professions (nurses, pharmacists, physicians, high school teachers, and police officers) are in healthcare. While these perceptions about healthcare

brand touch point/ brand contact point
any contact or interaction that reinforces an organization's brand or marketing message

professionals may give healthcare marketers a head start over marketers in other industries, healthcare marketers still need to make certain that their communications continuously build on and strengthen the relationships and loyalty among consumers, caregivers, and health organizations (Berkowitz 2011, 232):

relationship marketing
marketing communications that continuously build on and strengthen the relationships and loyalty among consumers and organizations

> The foundation of **relationship marketing** is to develop a strategy that shifts the organization's thinking from the individual transaction, such as getting the patient to come to the clinic, to a relationship focus of longer-term loyalty—defining the organization as the regular healthcare provider. Research has shown that relationship marketing is more effective in industries where relationships are more critical to customers. In no industry may this be more true than in healthcare.

Relationships must be two-way and mutually beneficial. Berkowitz (2011) is correct in that relationship marketing must alter an organization's thinking. The quote, however, is one-sided and describes only half of relationship building. The goal of relationship marketing must be more than just gaining the patient's loyalty; only the organization benefits from that loyalty. The organization must also be loyal to the patient; the patient must also benefit from the relationship by knowing that he will be treated with respect and honesty, that he will be safe, that care will be carefully provided and quality laden, that the people in the organization can be trusted to act ethically in any and all situations, and that he can count on the organization to truly care for his health and well-being.

That order is a tall one to fill. Health organizations can't, and probably shouldn't, be everything to everyone. But health marketing communications can go a long way toward building and maintaining this ideal relationship.

WHERE DID I READ THAT?

The types of communication channels and media available to healthcare marketers are far too numerous to be listed and individually analyzed in this text. Therefore, only the most recent—electronic media—is discussed in this chapter. Often people think of electronic social media as blogs, Facebook, YouTube, and Twitter, but there are a number of other electronic health communication venues.

electronic health record (EHR)
an electronic version of a patient's medical record

One that is often overlooked is the **electronic health record (EHR)**. Depending on the version and software, the EHR is an excellent mechanism for communication and information sharing between providers and their patients. By granting patients access to their EHRs, the provider/facility sends a clear message that healthcare is a shared endeavor and that it is not the sole owner of patients' information. While healthcare marketers themselves do not have access to patients' EHRs, they can make the important argument that access builds trust and enhances the relationship between the patient and the provider organization.

The Health Information Technology for Economic and Clinical Health (HITECH) Act requires providers to make meaningful use of EHRs, including giving patients electronic access to their health information and sending reminders to patients for follow-up or preventive care (Woodcock 2011). As long as organizations are required to meet the meaningful use criteria, healthcare marketers should leverage EHRs for health communications and relationship building.

Another electronic channel for health communication is an organization's or a physician's website. Not only can a well-built website provide basics such as contact and service information; it also can build message and branding consistency; put a face and personality on the health organization or provider; streamline scheduling; provide a wealth of health information via hot links, webcasts, and podcasts; and be a safe and trustworthy site for patient education. When a provider offers a website where patients can gather all the information they need about the facility, their appointments, and their health concerns in a one-stop-shopping experience, the provider has taken a huge step toward building relationships and loyalty. Conversely, a poorly designed website that makes information hard to find, requires the user to click 20 times to access anything of importance, and contains broken links is a relationship killer.

A 2011 study showed that most Americans would use secure online communications for their health and health-related activities, such as scheduling, requesting medication, obtaining lab results, completing forms, preregistering for care, and paying bills, if they were available (Lewis 2011). Because websites have become such a crucial and primary source of information and means of contact for patients and consumers, it is vital that marketing have primary control over them. Responsibility for the website should not be delegated to the organization's information technology (IT) department. All facets of the organization need to provide input, information, and materials. While construction of the website is the purview of the IT department, the marketing department needs to own and design the website; it is a core part of the organization's marketing strategy.

SUMMARY

Health marketing communication covers all the elements of basic communication but incorporates extra dimensions of education, service, and relationships. Internally and externally, an organization's marketing message and branding must be consistent. Everyone with the organization must see himself as part of the marketing team.

Chapter Questions

1. Why is listening such an important skill for healthcare marketers?
2. What is a communication channel? Name three and provide an example of effective healthcare marketing for each.
3. What is relationship marketing?
4. Why should everyone in an organization be a healthcare marketer?

Chapter Exercises

1. *Differentiation*

   Find three examples that differentiate health marketing communications from generic marketing communications. For each health marketing example, rate its communication as poor, average, good, or excellent and explain your rating.

2. *Prioritizing communication efforts*

   In this chapter's opening case, Kenji has quite a challenge ahead of him. If you were Kenji, how would you proceed? What would you do during your first four weeks on the job? Create a list of projects for Kenji and prioritize them. Identify the kinds of information Kenji needs for each project and whom he should include in each.

References

Berkowitz, E. N. 2011. *Essentials of Healthcare Marketing*. Sudbury, MA: Jones and Bartlett.

Bolon, D. S. 2005. "Comparing Mission Statement Content in For-Profit and Not-For-Profit Hospitals: Does Mission Really Matter?" *Hospital Topics* 83 (4): 2–9.

Gallup. 2012. "Honesty/Ethics in Professions." www.gallup.com/poll/1654/honesty-ethics-professions.aspx.

Lewis, N. 2011. "Majority of Patients Want Online Access to Doctors." *InformationWeek*
March 4. www.informationweek.com/news/healthcare/patient/229300352.

Woodcock, E. W. 2011. "Patient Engagement: Achieving Meaningful Use." White paper.
www.viterahealthcare.com/SiteCollectionDocuments/ARRA/White%20Paper%20-%20
Patient%20Engagement%20-%20Achieving%20Meaningful%20Use.pdf.

Yen, H. 2012. "Census: Minorities Now Surpass Whites in US Births." Associated Press (May
17). http://bigstory.ap.org/content/census-minorities-now-surpass-whites-us-births.

CHAPTER 11

CONFLICT MANAGEMENT

CASE STUDY: PRIMARY CARE MARKETING DILEMMA AND THE PODIATRIST STALEMATE

Joe Toniolo, office administrator at Riverside Podiatry in Pitt/Greene County, North Carolina, wanted the first-ever retreat of the four-podiatrist practice to go well. He read over the agenda one more time to make certain that the details were covered. He did not want the four hours to be filled with conversations that went nowhere. He wanted to end the stalemate among the podiatrists, help them resolve their conflicts, and present his marketing plan for the practice's future.

Joe felt that the practice could be busier and accommodate more patients. Even though he had followed through on his responsibility to direct marketing efforts, the practice had not seen any measurable **return on investment (ROI)**. Dr. Piede thought that advertising the practice via radio commercials, focusing on quality of care, and making appointments easier to schedule would bring in more patients. Dr. Martini disagreed, thinking that advertising would be a waste of money. The other two podiatrists thought that advertising was a good idea, but they wanted television to be included as a medium of delivery. The end result was frustration, stalemated conversations, and a tense work atmosphere for everyone in the office. Furthermore, their disagreements were interfering with Riverside Podiatry's ability to carry out its mission:

> Our mission is to provide the finest podiatric care and exceed your expectations. We realize that each patient—from the child to the elder, from the sports enthusiast to the couch potato—has individualized needs ranging from conservative care to surgical correction. We spend quality time with each patient to better understand your foot care needs and recommend the best course of treatment.

Joe knew this mission fit well with the practice. The four podiatrists really did want to exceed the expectations of their patients; they really did strive for excellence in practice. But the **conflict** and bickering over the lack of growth in the number of patients was having a negative effect on the office. The medical assistant had stopped by his office that morning to ask if he could do something about the tension and conflict among the podiatrists. "Really," she said, "you can feel the tension in the air. Joe, do something!"

Joe knew he had to do something to address the conflict among the physicians and the underlying problem that was adding fuel to the fire. He needed to improve his marketing efforts to get more patients to come to the practice. He hoped that the retreat would present a situation in which the podiatrists could handle conflicts in a responsible and fair way and focus on bringing attention back to what was good and in the interests of the practice. Thus, he had chosen to hold the retreat at Dr. Piede's vacation mountain home. The podiatrists and Joe would meet Saturday morning, and then the podiatrists would have the

return on investment (ROI)
a performance measure used to evaluate the success of initiatives that require an investment (in time, effort, and/or money)

conflict
a state of disharmony or lack of agreement between at least two parties over ideas, beliefs, or practices

rest of the weekend to enjoy the mountains with their families. Joe wanted the physicians to meet in an environment away from the office to make the retreat as stress-free as possible.

Joe checked off his agenda items. "Well," he thought, "I think I am ready as I'll ever be. Let's see if the others are ready to try, too."

Retreat Agenda Items

Item	Action
Icebreaker	• Outside retreat leader will direct the meeting and address points of conflict; outsider might get the physicians to respond professionally and keep them from arguing. • Joe will address other agenda items. • Present top-ten list of why we see podiatrists (a little humor to begin). • Discuss the importance of our mission (to center attendees' attention on the reason for the retreat).
Assessment	• North Carolina: on average, three podiatrists per 100,000 population.* • Pitt/Greene County: 180,000 people. • If Pitt/Greene County had the average number of podiatrists to population, the county would have six podiatrists. • Ten are practicing in the county, four more than the statewide average. • The county could support more than six, but ten presents a dilemma.
Mission of Riverside Podiatry (text proposed to be added to our mission is in italics)	*We work closely with primary care physicians and other specialists to ensure the most effective treatment plan.*

Strategy and objectives	1. Develop a brochure for distribution about Riverside Podiatry.
1. Market growth (find new markets; sell products to existing and new patients) 2. Branding (differentiate Riverside Podiatry)	2. Conduct a patient satisfaction survey. 3. Develop a referral-tracking and acknowledgment policy for referring physicians and patients who refer other patients. 4. Implement a referring provider direct-mail campaign. 5. Implement in-office dispensing of high-quality, podiatric products (e.g., lotions, creams, support shoes) at market price as convenience for patients. Package products in Riverside Podiatry personalized bags.
Defining task-related conflict—why it can be functional	Retreat leader will moderate discussion.
Target markets	1. General practitioners and family physicians, potential referrals in primary (Pitt/Greene County) and secondary (six adjacent counties that touch Pitt/Greene) service areas 2. Potential patients in primary and secondary service area
Expense budget	$7,500 for first quarter; budget to be a rolling budget and updated quarterly
Success measures and ROI	1. Increase number of patients served by 7% in 12 months. 2. Begin sales of podiatric products; break even within six months following implementation.
Conflict resolution	Retreat leader—resolution plan; focus on work and mission. Takeaways from the meeting to be highlighted.

Source: NCBPE (2010).

HEALTHCARE MARKETING AND CONFLICT MANAGEMENT

Managing clinics, practices, or departments requires teams of professionals—physicians, nurses, administrators, and allied health professionals—to work together so that patients receive the best care possible and their experiences exceed their expectations. However, when conflict exists, there are consequences in healthcare settings and delivery. In the case study, the medical assistant told Joe that she could feel the tension in the air, and she turned to him to do something about it.

Consider Joe's predicament. He is the administrator for a four-podiatrist practice and also serves as manager, human resources director, marketer, and administrative "fill-in" person (e.g., if the biller falls behind, Joe steps in to help; if the front-desk administrative assistant has to step away, he answers the phone). Joe likes working in the small practice environment as opposed to a larger clinic or hospital. He has come to really know the people with whom he works, and he likes the different responsibilities he has. If he had worked in a hospital, the marketing issues would have been delegated to the marketing and public relations department, for instance. But, just as working in a small practice has its benefits, it also has its disadvantages. He has to address conflict issues effectively while fulfilling all his other responsibilities.

No matter where he might have worked, conflict would have been inevitable. People have conflicting views over what should be done and how it should be done, and people have interpersonal differences. Conflict is a "natural outcome of human interaction" (Rahim 2010, 1):

> When two or more social entities (i.e., individuals, groups, organizations, and nations) come in contact with one another in attaining their objectives, their relationships may become incompatible or inconsistent. Relationships among such entities may become inconsistent when two or more of them desire a similar resource that is in short supply; when they have partially exclusive behavioral preferences regarding their joint action; or when they have different attitudes, values, beliefs, and skills.

FUNCTIONAL AND DYSFUNCTIONAL CONFLICT

task conflict
disagreement over the content of decisions relating to a particular task

In Joe's case, the conflict seems to have emerged because the podiatrists have differing opinions regarding how to best address the flat patient growth (i.e., task conflict). Karen Jehn (1997, 1995), professor of management at the University of Melbourne, defined three types of conflict:

relationship conflict
disagreement over personal issues; interpersonal differences

1. **Task conflict** is disagreement about the content of decisions related to a particular task.

2. **Relationship conflict** results when at least two people differ about non-work-related behavior. This type of conflict can be poison to an organization's goals.

If the professionals are focused on interpersonal struggles, their ability to work together on behalf of the task at hand is diminished.

3. **Process conflict** is disagreement over the delegation of workload—that is, conflict arises because there is disagreement about who is responsible for what task.

process conflict
disagreement over workload delegation

Theodore Caplow (1983), commonwealth professor emeritus of sociology at the University of Virginia, stated that in conflicts among staff members of differing or similar positions, authority matters—that is, it is important to note whether the conflict has arisen from a personal feud among equally ranked members or from persecution of a subordinate by his or her superior (more on this subject is presented in the next section).

Past research indicates that relationship conflict is more likely than the other two types of conflict to be detrimental to an organization because the parties are spending more time antagonizing and distrusting each other than focusing on work solutions (Jehn and Mannix 2001). Consequences of **dysfunctional conflict** include wasted time (Suppiah and Rose 2006) and poor individual well-being (e.g., feeling burned out, lacking energy) (De Dreu, van Dierendonck, and Dijkstra 2004). Unless handled expertly, relationship conflict is dysfunctional. If Joe were dealing with a relationship conflict (e.g., two of the podiatrists distrusted and disliked each other), little headway would be made on resolving their issues for the benefit of the practice.

dysfunctional conflict
conflict that may contribute to a decline in work performance

When conflict emerges, however, it may not be all negative. While the work environment is tense, the presence of conflict has inspired Joe to seriously consider and develop the upcoming retreat to present his plan for addressing the underlying problem—increasing marketing efforts to address the low patient census. Thus, the differences among the podiatrists could be considered **functional conflict** because the situation is forcing Joe to think strategically and creatively and present a rational marketing solution that may work for the benefit of the practice.

functional conflict
conflict that may contribute to positive work performance

Howard Guttman, a prominent management consultant, identified conflict management as a core competency for human resources managers—one of Joe's roles in the practice. Conflict may create devastating problems, but it does not have to do so. The outcome is dependent on how the conflict is managed (Guttman 2009, 33).

RESPONSES TO CONFLICT

Let us first address the handling of relationship conflict. As mentioned earlier, Caplow (1983) distinguished between persons of similar rank and persons of differing rank and asserted that the positioning of employees matters. When an administrator must address relationship conflict that has emerged from the persecution of a subordinate by his or her superior, Caplow (1983) recommended that a neutral third party be brought in so that all parties are treated ethically and with justice.

As elaborated in Chapter 4, John Rawls introduced the concept of procedural justice as the adoption of a fair procedure to help bring about an equitable outcome. He used the simple process of cake slice allocation to exemplify procedural justice. If one person is told to cut a cake and let others choose their slices first, the person will cut equally sized slices so that he is assured an equal share (Rawls 1971, 84). Hence, a fair process helps bring about a fair outcome. Healthcare marketing managers often make decisions in which fairness plays a role because they are involved with how employees are treated. By bringing in a neutral party, the healthcare marketing manager is not siding with one side or the other; rather, issues will be identified and a resolution will be proposed through a process that employees will perceive as fair. Hospitals, for example, have grievance committees—typically housed in a separate human resources department—that address such actions. Nonetheless, Joe works in a physician practice and acts as the human resources grievance representative as well as the healthcare marketing manager.

As elaborated earlier, Caplow (1983) noted that authority matters. However, when relationship conflict emerges between two equally ranked parties, the healthcare marketing manager is facing a situation in which rational discussion may not be effective. Both parties involved in the conflict are focused on interpersonal emotions. For instance, Riverside Podiatry employs one front-desk administrative assistant and one medical assistant, both highly valued employees. For the sake of this example, let us propose that the two had a dispute. The medical assistant dislikes the way the administrative assistant speaks to others in the office, including patients. She is known to use words such as *sugar, honey*, and *sweetie-pie*. She sees nothing wrong with these titles because she thinks they are endearing words and let others know that she cares about them. When asked to stop by the medical assistant, she refused and replied that it was just the way she talked. The conflict has grown to the status of a feud, and both parties' behavior at work has been negative as a result. It is interfering with patient flow and daily operations of the practice and has created an unpleasant environment for the nurses and for Joe. As the administrator, Joe needs to solve the dilemma while not encouraging one or the other to quit (remember, they are both highly valued). Speaking with each one individually has not helped; both are entrenched in the belief that they are right and the other is a troublemaker. Neither is willing to consider the other's position. Speaking with them collaboratively has not helped either; they've only became more deeply entrenched in their positions and refuse to compromise or problem-solve.

Caplow (1983, 152) proposed that the best strategy for resolving such a feud is for the administrator to take one side or the other. The outcome of taking such a stance is threefold. First, others in the practice need not get involved because the one supported by Joe (the winner) no longer needs others to support her stance. It also reduces the need for others in the practice to support the other employee (the loser). Second, the loser may find saving face and ending the feud more appealing now that the administrator has sided with the other party. Last and most important, the danger that both will quit is diminished.

The winner no longer has a motive to quit. She has Joe's support. The loser is less likely to leave than she would have been if the feud had been allowed to continue, but some risk of leaving is still present. Nonetheless, the feud ends, and at least one valued employee, if not both, remains.

Modes of response to conflict have been classified into five types: (1) withdrawing or avoiding; (2) smoothing, obliging, or accommodating; (3) compromising or sharing; (4) forcing or dominating; and (5) problem solving or integrating (Blake and Mouton 1964; Chou and Yeh 2007; Johansen 2012). While the terms have changed over time, the emphasis remains on how the conflict may be managed effectively so that staff members may do their work well. Let's look at some examples of how each of these response modes might play out in the case study:

1. *Withdrawing or avoiding:* Joe refuses to address the situation between the medical assistant and front-desk administrative assistant. Both employees are entrenched in their positions, and the conflict grows.

2. *Smoothing, obliging, or accommodating:* Joe asks the medical assistant to consider the administrative assistant's position and just accept it.

3. *Compromising or sharing:* Joe looks for middle ground and asks them both to consider how they could address the issue and be comfortable with the resolution.

4. *Forcing or dominating:* Joe takes a stand and sides with one or the other.

5. *Problem solving or integrating:* Joe involves the medical assistant and front-desk administrative assistant and looks for a resolution. Creative problem solving and empowerment of the medical assistant and front-desk administrative assistant could have resulted from speaking with them collaboratively, but as noted earlier, this approach was to no avail.

Key to the discussion about what healthcare marketing managers may consider as they address relationship conflict is a focus on problem solving, not solving the interpersonal conflict. The same is true when dealing with process or task conflict. Attention should be given to problem solving, not to the dispute itself. Past research has shown the problem-solving mode of response to conflict is usually more effective than the other responses (Blake and Mouton 1964; Chou and Yeh 2007; Montoya-Weiss, Massey, and Song 2001). Nonetheless, the situation may encourage adoption of another mode of response. Joe tried integration and problem solving by communicating with the parties separately and together. When that failed, he shifted to dominating and took a side. Thus, at times, one mode of conflict management may be more appropriate than another, given the specifics of the situation.

HEALTHCARE MARKETERS AS CRITICAL THINKERS AND CREATIVE PROBLEM SOLVERS

The concepts that guide conflict management help healthcare marketing managers to serve as critical thinkers and creative problem solvers. As a healthcare administrator in a small practice who "wears many hats," Joe has frameworks that he may refer to as he fulfills his responsibilities. First and foremost, as a critical thinker, Joe must define the problem correctly. The dilemma in the case study—underproduction and the need to increase the number of patients—needs to be addressed. And this dilemma is what his retreat agenda attempts to address by adopting a problem-solving or an integrating response.

Joe plans to present market demographics and identify market need for podiatric services in the county area by population (see the assessment section in his list of agenda items at the beginning of the chapter). The county is oversaturated—that is, more podiatrists than needed are practicing in the area. Bringing this situation to the podiatrists' attention is an important step for Joe to take. The podiatrists need to understand what is contributing to their lower-than-desired production.

Joe also plans to review the mission of Riverside Podiatry and recommend that the podiatrists consider adding one sentence to it (see the mission section in his list of agenda items). Reviewing the mission will help center the podiatrists' attention on the reasons for the retreat—their work and practice—and may help to foster solidarity among them as they work to identify target markets and ways to increase the number of patients.

Joe plans to encourage the podiatrists to consider the development of relationship marketing with a targeted market segment: referring physicians (i.e., primary care physicians). *Relationship marketing* is defined as "proactively creating, developing and maintaining committed, interactive and profitable exchanges with selected customers [partners] over time" (Harker 1999, 16). (See Chapter 10 for a discussion of relationship marketing.) Particularly in North Carolina, which ranked 13th among the states for highest prevalence of adult diabetes in 2012 (see www.ncdiabetes.org), proper foot care is important because diabetes may impair circulation in the legs and feet and/or cause a loss of nerve function in these areas. Primary care physicians may encourage their patients (especially patients with diabetes) to seek specialist attention for foot care. Hence, working closely with primary care physicians on behalf of their patients promotes better healthcare. Moreover, by following up with primary care physicians and providing them with feedback about the patients they referred to Riverside Podiatry, the podiatrists reinforce to the physicians that Riverside Podiatry indeed provides excellent care, and the primary care physicians are likely to refer their patients to Riverside again.

Joe wants the podiatrists to support his proposal to focus on building long-term bonds between the practice and the referring physicians as one way to address the lower-than-desired production. And, by getting the podiatrists to focus together on reasonable solutions, express buy-in, and take ownership of the issue at hand, Joe may help reduce/eliminate the conflict that has emerged between them.

Joe also is planning to strategically address areas outside of Pitt/Greene County to expand Riverside's outreach to potential referring physicians in surrounding counties. Patients might drive 20 to 30 minutes more to see a podiatrist at Riverside instead of one in their immediate area for the same reasons just described: Family physicians in surrounding counties will know that their patients will receive excellent care and that the podiatrist will not only keep them informed about their patients via follow-up but also partner with them regarding treatment plans. Long-term relationships will emerge; Riverside will experience **market growth** because of the increase in patients, and the podiatrists can do what they do best—provide excellent specialty care.

market growth
increase in demand for services provided or products sold

Joe will introduce another market growth strategy as well—the sale of foot care products to existing and new patients. It is becoming more common for healthcare providers to offer products for sale in their offices. The American Dental Association addressed the marketing/sale of products in dental offices in 1999, emphasizing that dentists who engage in the sale of dental products (e.g., electronic toothbrushes, teeth-whitening kits) must "take care not to exploit the trust" of their patients (ADA 1999, 2). Joe will propose that the podiatrists consider following this model. Stocking the office with certain products known for their excellence can provide another revenue source for the practice. This service is one way to build long-term relationships with patients; it offers convenience and expert advice regarding foot care products.

Moreover, Joe will propose that the podiatrists consider differentiating Riverside Podiatry via new **branding** efforts. *Branding* is defined as "establishing efficient, choice-shaping association with the brand name" (Walvis 2008, 180). Joe's aim, therefore, is to have referring physicians and patients have positive choice-shaping associations with Riverside Podiatry. To this end, providing excellent care, exceeding patients' expectations, and working closely with referring physicians will factor into establishing such positive associations with Riverside Podiatry.

branding
establishing positive associations with an organization in the minds of customers (In healthcare, customers are patients, physicians, and the public.)

The retreat that Joe has planned does not center on solving the doctors' conflicts. Rather, Joe is focused on managing conflict via problem solving and reinforcement of the organization's mission. He is proposing marketing initiatives that (he hopes) will provide effective resolution to the underlying issue that helped to bring about the conflict in the first place. Although research indicates that conflict has adverse effects in the workplace, it is important for marketing managers to recognize that positive outcomes may occur if the conflict is managed effectively. It might be frustrating and stressful to work in an environment of conflict, but conflict is inevitable. To manage the conflict as best as possible, marketing managers should be mindful of mission and remain focused on their ability to problem-solve.

CHAPTER QUESTIONS

1. Joe hired an outside leader to direct the retreat. Why did he think that the presence of an outsider might deflect conflict? Consider in your answer the significance of holding the retreat away from the office and the specific agenda items Joe planned with the outside leader.

2. Recall from your school, work, or volunteer experiences an episode in which relationship conflict emerged between two equally ranked parties. How was the conflict resolved? Was it resolved successfully? What is your assessment of Caplow's (1983) proposal that one take one side or the other? How might that approach have worked in the conflict you recalled?

3. Joe is planning to introduce two strategies to increase the patient census at Riverside Podiatry: finding new markets (i.e., gaining referrals from physicians in surrounding counties) and selling products to patients. How would you measure the success of each strategy?

CHAPTER EXERCISES

1. *Communicating to the referring physicians about Phoenix Cardiac Surgery*

In April 2012, the investigation of Phoenix Cardiac Surgery, P.C. (www .phoenixcardiacsurgery.com) by the US Department of Health and Human Services Office for Civil Rights ended with Phoenix's agreement to implement a corrective plan of action and pay a $100,000 fine. Phoenix had been posting clinical and surgical appointments on a publicly accessible, Internet-based calendar for more than ten years (Larose and Gold 2012). It is a violation of HIPAA not to protect the privacy of patients' personal health information.

For this exercise, assume you are Phoenix Cardiac Surgery's practice administrator. You wear many hats in your job. You are responsible for operations management, marketing, human resources, and more. You do what needs to be done to keep the practice operating smoothly so that the surgeons can attend to their patients. The five surgeons in the practice perform cardiac and thoracic surgery as well as provide varicose vein treatment.

Some patients are self-referred, but a significant portion of patients comes from referrals from family practice physicians. You know that the news about your HIPAA violation and the fines and corrective plan of action may have a negative effect on referrals from outside stakeholders (i.e., referring physicians).

With the concept of relationship marketing in mind, propose a plan to mitigate the negative effects of the HIPAA violation and focus on rebranding Phoenix Cardiac Surgery as the practice that referring physicians have confidence in to provide excellent patient care.

2. *Market growth via new products for existing and new patients*

You are the director of communications for the Monmart Indiana Regional Medical Center (MIRMC). The executive director has asked you to investigate whether it is a good idea for MIRMC to increase its revenue line by selling cookbooks at its health promotion events. She is envisioning MIRMC's sale of cookbooks like Mayo Clinic's sale of diet books, but she is uncertain if selling books (1) is ethical and (2) an effective way to increase revenue while providing excellence in healthcare services to the community. She knows that it will be a hard sell to get some of the board members to go along with the idea. To prevent unnecessary conflict, she has asked you to prepare a two-page (double-spaced) summary that supports or does not support market growth via the selling of cookbooks at MIRMC's health promotion events.

REFERENCES

American Dental Association (ADA). 1999. "Marketing or Sale of Products or Procedures." Report and advisory opinion of the Council on Ethics, Bylaws and Judicial Affairs. Revised in June. www.ada.org/files/Final_Report_on_Adv_Op_5_D_2_7-28-99-S.pdf.

Blake, R., and J. Mouton. 1964. *The Managerial Grid: Key Orientations for Achieving Production Through People*. Houston, TX: Gulf Publishing Company.

Caplow, T. 1983. *Managing an Organization*, second edition. New York: Holt, Rinehart, and Winston.

Chou, H., and Y. Yeh. 2007. "Conflict, Conflict Management, and Performance in ERP Teams." *Social Behavior and Personality* 35 (8): 1035–48.

De Dreu, C. K. W., D. van Dierendonck, and M. T. M. Dijkstra. 2004. "Conflict at Work and Individual Well-Being." *International Journal of Conflict Management* 15 (1): 6–26.

Guttman, H. M. 2009. "Conflict Management as a Core Competency for HR Professionals." *People & Strategy* 32 (1): 33–39.

Harker, J. 1999. "Relationship Marketing Defined? An Examination of Current Relationship Marketing Definitions." *Marketing Intelligence & Planning* 17 (1): 13–20.

Jehn, K. A. 1997. "A Qualitative Analysis of Conflict Types and Dimensions in Organizational Groups." *Administrative Science Quarterly* 42 (3): 530–57.

————. 1995. "A Multimethod Examination of the Benefits and Detriments of Intragroup Conflict." *Administrative Science Quarterly* 40 (2): 256–82.

Jehn, K. A., and E. A. Mannix. 2001. "The Dynamic Nature of Conflict: A Longitudinal Study of Intragroup Conflict and Group Performance." *Academy of Management Journal* 44 (2): 238–51.

Johansen, M. 2012. "Keeping the Peace: Conflict Management Strategies for Nurse Managers." *Nursing Management* 18 (9): 50–54.

Larose, C., and K. Gold, for Mintz Levin. 2012. "The Rising Cost of HIPAA Violations: $100,000 Fine Levied on Physician Group." *JD Supra Law News* (April 20).

Montoya-Weiss, M., A. Massey, and M. Song. 2001. "Getting It Together: Temporal Coordination and Conflict Management in Global Virtual Teams." *Academy of Management Journal* 44 (6): 1251–62.

North Carolina Board of Podiatry Examiners (NCBPE). 2010. "Podiatrists per 10,000 Population, North Carolina, 2010." http://ncbpe.org/sites/default/files/2010%20data%20 -%20DPMs%20per%2010K%20pop.pdf.

Rahim, M. 2010. *Managing Conflict in Organizations*. Piscataway, NJ: Transaction Publishers.

Rawls, J. 1971. *A Theory of Justice*. Cambridge, MA: Belknap Press.

Suppiah, W., and R. Rose. 2006. "A Competence-Based View to Conflict Management." *American Journal of Applied Sciences* 3 (7): 1905–909.

Walvis, T. 2008. "Three Laws of Branding: Neuroscientific Foundations of Effective Brand Building." *Brand Management* 16 (3): 176–94.

CHAPTER 12

TEAMWORK AND LEADERSHIP

After studying this chapter, you will be able to

➤ describe the qualities of effective teams,

➤ build effective teams,

➤ recognize how leadership characteristics apply to marketing, and

➤ discuss the role and functions of the marketing manager.

CASE STUDY: OPPORTUNITIES AND CHALLENGES

Inez Montero had been the director of marketing at St. Patricia's Hospital for almost six months. St. Pat's was a community-owned hospital with 130 acute care beds, located in a city of approximately 120,000 people. The city had recently been hard hit by recession; two large, local employers had gone out of business, and many people were unemployed and without health insurance. Inez had a degree in healthcare administration with a minor in marketing and had started working at St. Pat's four years ago as one of the marketing staff. She had a natural aptitude for marketing, for understanding healthcare, and for turning a phrase. In addition, she worked easily with others on the marketing team, clinicians, and other hospital managers. She had steadily progressed up the ladder from the lowest staff position to marketing team coordinator. When the position of marketing director opened up, she applied and got it.

St. Pat's was the only acute care hospital in the area but had been struggling; its physical plant was getting old, and people in the community often referred to the hospital as "old St. Pat's." It had recently installed its first electronic medical record system, but the new technology was not well received among the physicians and nurses; in fact, many of the clinicians refused to use it. The hospital's efforts to get a website and new computerized admissions process up and running also had been unsuccessful. Two new urgent care clinics had opened in the area, and St. Pat's cardiologists had recently formed a new specialty group practice, which was offering many of the tests and less invasive procedures that had always been performed at St. Pat's. The region was becoming flooded with billboards, radio spots, flyers, and other advertisements touting these new patient care venues.

St. Pat's had always hired Keller Public Relations, an outside firm, to handle all of its public events and promotions for those events. Over the years, Inez had little if any interaction with Keller PR herself, but from the rest of the marketing department's point of view, Keller PR was a constant problem and source of great frustration. Now that Inez was in charge, St. Pat's CEO had decided to end the hospital's relationship with Keller PR and merge all the PR functions into Inez's marketing department. Inez had been pleased by this expansion of her responsibilities until she realized that, because Keller PR had always been completely in charge of all of St. Pat's PR, nobody on her staff had any real PR expertise. Thankfully, the CEO had agreed that Inez should hire a PR team leader.

Many people applied for the new position, but few of them were qualified. The one truly qualified applicant, Gary Grafenstein, was the second in command at Keller PR. When Inez and her hiring team interviewed Gary, she found him to be bright, personable, and brimming with great ideas; he seemed to be a true team player. And because he had worked on St. Pat's PR while at Keller PR, he already knew the organization and would be able to hit the pavement running. Even though the hiring committee agreed that he was by far the best applicant (indeed he was the only applicant they were seriously considering), Inez worried about how the people in her department would receive Gary—an employee from the firm they hated—particularly as a team leader. Her hiring committee was evenly divided; two wanted to hire him and two did not. It looked like the decision was up to Inez. She decided to think about it over the weekend and announce her decision Monday morning.

Late Sunday evening, Inez received an e-mail from her CEO, saying that he had just come up with a brilliant idea for St. Pat's. He was going to officially change their facility's name from St. Patricia's Hospital to St. Patricia's Medical Center. He had contacted the board over the weekend, and all of the board members had agreed. The new name would reenergize St. Pat's image and help move St. Pat's into a new era. He already had St. Pat's in-house lawyer putting together the legal papers to officially change the name.

For Inez, this change was an incredible opportunity to display her team-building, leadership, and marketing skills; every single aspect of St. Pat's marketing and PR would need to be reevaluated and updated to reflect the new name. Under her leadership and direction, her marketing department would be able to create and redesign everything. She thought she might even design a new organizational logo. The project was truly exciting!

TEAMWORK AND LEADERSHIP

Healthcare marketing is a **team-centered** activity. As the complexity of the healthcare environment increases, the need for professional exchange, purposeful interaction, and collaboration is growing along with it. "The pressures for cost control and value creation in healthcare delivery, for maximizing productivity, and for improving quality through integration and coordination are strong and increasing" (Begun, White, and Mosser 2011, 120). The need to provide good information and marketing messages about the ever-amazing growth in services, treatments, and delivery options requires the skills, knowledge, and experience of a wide range of clinical and nonclinical staff (Fletcher 2008). Thus, health marketers need to be able to work with the entire spectrum of their healthcare colleagues.

HEALTHCARE MARKETING TEAMS

Teamwork is much more than simply putting a group of people together to work on a task. Some of the factors that go into developing effective teams are attitudes, behaviors, and knowledge. **Attitudes** are individuals' internal states, which affect a team's ability to interact and work together. **Behaviors** are the application of skills, actions, and abilities necessary to accomplish the work, and **knowledge** refers to the prior experiences and understandings that team members bring to the task at hand and that guide the team's work (Shuffler, Granados, and Salas 2011).

Regardless of industry or setting, teams almost always go through specific stages of development (Cellucci and Wiggins 2009, 87):

---

team-centered
characterized by purposeful exchange, interaction, and collaboration along a spectrum of knowledgeable professionals

attitudes
individuals' internal states, which affect a team's ability to work together

behaviors
the application of skills, actions, and abilities necessary to accomplish the work

knowledge
prior experiences and understandings that team members bring to the task at hand and that guide the team's work

1. **Forming:** Members are given their charge and learn the purpose of the team.

2. **Storming:** As members learn about each other, conflict and emotional issues may arise.

3. **Norming:** Members agree on working styles and processes, conflict decreases, and group cohesiveness develops.

4. **Performing:** Members engage in and complete the team's work and achieve the team's purpose.

5. **Adjourning:** Members review outcomes and disengage from the team.

Assembling an effective marketing team in healthcare, however, has its own challenges. Healthcare is complex and emotional. Members of the health marketing team must not only understand marketing; they must also be sensitive to its role in healthcare. They must understand the complexity of healthcare's innumerable products, treatments, venues, payment mechanisms, and care providers. Because so many professionals and disciplines are involved in the delivery of care and thus contribute knowledge and information for the production and distribution of the healthcare marketing message, there is bound to be disagreement about what the message should be and how it should be disseminated. On top of that, many people inside healthcare still believe that marketing is only about pressure and selling, and this perception can cause great concern and dissonance among the health professionals contributing information to the message. A key component of team building is trust (Clark, Kokko, and White 2012, 928):

> You can have all the vision, mission, expectations, policies, and procedures in the world; without trust, your team . . . is going nowhere. Trust is the important leadership virtue that must exist if a team is going to function to meet its challenges and opportunities.

Healthcare is hierarchical and political, with large knowledge and power gaps among the disciplines; the members of the marketing team must be able to tactfully and successfully navigate among health professionals while still achieving the team's purpose and goals, and that takes leadership.

LEADERSHIP

Leadership is one of those things that people talk about but have a hard time defining. Even if people can't easily define it, they think they know it when they see it. However, leadership can be defined, and it can be learned. There are many ways to think about

forming
the first stage of teamwork; members are given their charge and learn the purpose of the team

storming
the second stage of teamwork; as members learn about each other, conflict and emotional issues may arise

norming
the third, or middle, stage of teamwork; members agree on working styles and processes, conflict decreases, and group cohesiveness develops

performing
the fourth stage of teamwork; members engage in and complete the team's work and achieve the team's purpose

adjourning
the final stage of teamwork; members review outcomes and disengage from the team

leadership. Is leadership a trait, a dimension of personality that one is born with and influences what one does? Or is it a skill or competency? Could it be a behavior? Finally, could it also be a relationship? Can one be a leader if there are no followers?

All of these questions suggest ways to think about leadership. However, six leadership traits have direct application in marketing: (1) intelligence, (2) confidence, (3) charisma, (4) determination, (5) sociability, and (6) integrity (Northouse 2009).

Intelligence in this sense is not necessarily IQ. It is being knowledgeable about the discipline of marketing and about the products the health marketer is communicating. It includes language skills, reasoning ability, and an understanding about what is going on inside and outside the organization. It is knowing what needs to be done to successfully spread the marketing message and knowing how to fine-tune it to niches and segments appropriately.

Confidence builds on this foundation of knowledge and comes from understanding one's own abilities and skills. Confidence is not arrogance. It comes from being consciously competent— knowing not only what marketing techniques, channels, and messages work but also why they work in specific situations. Confidence comes from knowing that one can achieve one's goals and from constantly practicing and honing skills.

Charisma is an essential leadership characteristic for health marketers to have but is often overlooked. Having charisma does not just mean being well liked and popular. Charismatic leaders are role models and are inspiring. Charisma is an important facet of marketing, perhaps even more so when one is working to go beyond simply selling or creating demand for a product. When a health marketer is working to create a stellar reputation and a relationship between his organization and the public, having charisma's strong values and ability to attract and maintain loyalty is key.

Determination is a part of all marketing. Conventional wisdom says that a person needs to hear a message at least seven times before he absorbs and internalizes it. But determination is not redundancy; it is knowing where the message needs to go, what outcomes are desired, and how to find a number of interesting and engaging ways to get it there. Determination involves initiative, persistence, and drive. It means staying focused and staying the course. It is insisting on alignment and consistency between all marketing endeavors and the organization's mission, vision, and goals.

Some marketers seem to think that marketing is all about **sociability**—big campaign kickoffs, PR events, giveaways, and parties. Without a doubt, these kinds of events are important. In healthcare, events and items such as free blood pressure checks, bandages with a hospital's logo, and refrigerator magnets abound. These sorts of things are all excellent ways to support and promote an organization's brand and message. But too often they are one-shot deals, a lot of sizzle with little or no substance behind them. For healthcare marketers, sociability must go beyond the sizzle and focus on building professional relationships. Because of the life-or-death nature of healthcare and because everything health organizations do is intrinsically emotion laden and personal, health marketing leaders must

intelligence
being knowledgeable about the discipline of marketing and about the products the health marketer is communicating

confidence
recognition of one's own abilities and skills; the state of being consciously competent

charisma
a quality of inspiring role models that comes from having strong, visible values and an ability to attract and maintain loyalty

determination
initiative, persistence, and drive; staying focused and staying the course

sociability
the ability to build and maintain appropriate and productive professional relationships

demonstrate deep and enduring sensitivity and care in all of their messages and communications, all of which are the very foundation of sociability.

All of the leadership traits and characteristics just discussed must be firmly rooted in **integrity**. Everyone, from physicians to patients, views health marketing with the eyes of a skeptic. If an organization posts its mission and vision on its walls, it must visibly live them. If its marketing messages talk about caring and quality, the organization must deliver 100 percent on those messages. If a marketer's colleagues don't believe that she is sincere about the campaigns she is proposing and promoting, it will be difficult to convince them to participate and collaborate. If a marketer comes across as slick and uncaring, his marketing messages will be suspect and will not only be ignored; they will also be despised. In an industry such as healthcare, where the competition is fierce and it is perceived that organizations will do or say almost anything to attract patients and to make a profit, personal integrity, and the integrity of one's messages, is paramount.

Finally, Peter Drucker (introduced in Chapter 3 of this book) provides a way to think about leaders that easily complements the previous discussion. Drucker (as cited by Flaherty 1999) proposed that a leader's job includes the following four components:

1. *Purpose:* "[The] capacity to get the right things done . . . a clear sense of mission . . . applying talent and intelligence to the right things" (Flaherty 1999, 282)

2. *Performance:* "The consistent ability to produce quantitative and qualitative results over a long period of time in a variety of assignments" (Flaherty 1999, 283)

3. *Motivation:* "Having positive feelings toward the job and possessing a sense of pride about the products and services of the corporation . . . the job . . . [is] the avenue to self-development" (Flaherty 1999, 283)

4. *Practice:* "In viewing the job as a learning process, Drucker suggested that the key to effectiveness was practice. And as with any practice, job practice did not come automatically but could be acquired through constant learning. This meant the chief challenge for managing the job was to enable ordinary people to do extraordinary things. . . . 'Effectiveness . . . is a habit; that is, a complex of practices'" (Drucker 1993, 23; Flaherty 1999, 284–85).

MANAGING THE MARKETING DEPARTMENT

It is the job of all managers to plan, organize, direct, and control; a marketing manager's job is no different. In **planning**, managers define goals and the specific tasks and actions necessary to achieving these goals. The manager then proceeds by building and **organizing**

integrity
the quality of being whole, sincere, and authentic

planning
defining goals and the specific tasks and actions necessary to achieving them

organizing
scheduling, team building, delegating, assigning projects and work, and ensuring staff have adequate resources to complete their work

directing

motivating, influencing, and ensuring effective and timely implementation and completion of tasks; communicating goals, deadlines, and desired outcomes

her staff to undertake the tasks by scheduling, forming teams, delegating, and assigning projects and work. She communicates goals, deadlines, and desired outcomes. **Directing** refers to motivating and influencing one's staff to ensure effective and timely implementation and completion of the tasks. Directing might include ongoing communications, exchange of information, updates, and meetings to ensure that tasks and projects are successfully moving forward. Last, **controlling** involves monitoring and evaluating the plan, the tasks, and completion of the tasks. The manager determines the effectiveness of the project and gets tasks back on track if needed. Controlling is an ongoing responsibility as the work unfurls as well as after the tasks have been completed.

controlling

monitoring and evaluating the plan, the tasks, and completion of the tasks and the project

Marketing managers may work under a director of marketing or, depending on the size and structure of the organization, under the chief operating officer or the CEO. In the case of a physician group practice, marketing managers may report directly to the practice owner(s). Drucker (1974, 465) said, "The first managerial skill is . . . effective decisions." The authors of this book carry this quote to its natural extension in the context of marketing management: The first managerial skill is effective decisions in planning, organizing, directing, and controlling the health marketing function.

CONCLUSION

Whether a marketing manager is part of a large corporate healthcare system or the solo marketing and PR person in a small office, he must have a deep and thorough understanding of healthcare and the healthcare products he is sharing in his marketing message. He must be able to work with others in his organization, build and work on teams, assume the leadership role, and become proficient in the skills of a manager.

CHAPTER QUESTIONS

1. Why is it so important that healthcare marketing be a team-centered function?
2. Why is trust such an important component of team building in healthcare?
3. Which of the six leadership traits discussed in this chapter is the most important for a healthcare marketing team leader to master? Why?

CHAPTER EXERCISES

1. *Introducing Gary as the PR team leader*

   In this chapter's opening case, Inez is faced with challenges and opportunities. Being sensitive to the fact that Gary not only comes from Keller PR but also was second in command there, and using the three factors that characterize effective teams (attitudes, behaviors, and knowledge) as your framework, suggest a plan for Inez for introducing Gary as the department's new PR team leader, mentoring him, and ensuring his success.

2. *Demonstrating leadership for the team*

   While changing St. Pat's name from "hospital" to "medical center" may seem to be simply a cosmetic word change, Inez has an opportunity to completely revamp St. Pat's image and brand. She must demonstrate all six leadership traits discussed in this chapter (intelligence, confidence, charisma, determination, sociability, and integrity) as she works to ensure positive communications, a positive image, and positive brand outcomes. For each leadership trait, describe specific activities for Inez to engage in that would concretely demonstrate her leadership.

3. *What's in a name?*

   St. Pat's has been struggling with its image. The economic times are not good, and competition for revenue and patients is becoming intense. Suggest three ways to leverage St. Pat's name change to address these challenges.

REFERENCES

Begun, J. W., K. R. White, and G. Mosser. 2011. "Interprofessional Care Teams: The Role of the Healthcare Administrator." *Journal of Interprofessional Care* 25 (2): 119–23.

Cellucci, L. W., and C. Wiggins. 2009. *Essential Techniques for Healthcare Managers*. Chicago: Health Administration Press.

Clark, T., H. Kokko, and S. J. White. 2012. "Trust: An Essential Element of Leaders and Managers." *American Journal of Health-System Pharmacy* 69 (11): 928–30.

Drucker, P. F. 1993. *The Effective Executive*. New York: HarperBusiness.

———. 1974. *Management: Tasks, Responsibilities, Practices*. New York: Harper and Row.

Flaherty, J. 1999. *Peter Drucker: Shaping the Managerial Mind: How the World's Foremost Management Thinker Crafted the Essentials of Business Success.* San Francisco: Jossey-Bass.

Fletcher, M. 2008. "Multi-Disciplinary Team Working: Building and Using the Team." *Practice Nurse* 35 (12): 42–47.

Northouse, P. G. 2009. *Introduction to Leadership: Concepts and Practice.* Thousand Oaks, CA: Sage.

Shuffler, M. L., D. D. Granados, and E. Salas. 2011. "There's a Science for That: Team Development Interventions in Organizations." *Current Directions in Psychological Science* 20 (6): 365–72.

PART IV

STRATEGIC ACTIONS OF THE HEALTHCARE MARKETER

This case is descriptive rather than decision oriented and requires analysis to understand the dynamics of the situation but does not require any recommendations for action to be made. It profiles various elements of a model healthcare organization and invites students to consider a number of questions and topics addressed in the text and brought to light in the story of Intermountain Healthcare.

Information for this case was derived from Intermountain's website at www.intermount ainhealthcare.org.

INTRODUCTION

After its founding in 1975, Salt Lake City, Utah–based Intermountain Healthcare evolved from 15 loosely affiliated not-for-profit hospitals in Utah, Idaho, and Wyoming to a fully integrated healthcare delivery system widely recognized as one of the finest healthcare organizations in the world.

COMPANY OVERVIEW

Through the years, Intermountain came to own and operate 22 hospitals, 185 clinics, and various health insurance plans from SelectHealth and brought together more than 1,000 physicians and clinicians in the Intermountain Medical Group. Intermountain Healthcare was the largest healthcare provider in the Intermountain West, with more than 33,000 employees serving the healthcare needs of Utah and southeastern Idaho residents. (A numerical overview of Intermountain Healthcare is provided in Exhibit 1.) Excellent clinical care was the basis of Intermountain's mission and the organization's greatest concern. Whether through its high-tech/high-touch clinical programs or by improving the treatment of certain chronic diseases, all three parts of Intermountain Healthcare (i.e., hospitals, medical group, and insurance plans) contributed in essential ways to the sharing of best medical practices—and raising the standards of clinical excellence.

EXHIBIT 1

Intermountain Healthcare by the Numbers (2012)

Charity cases/care	239,195/$252 million
Hospitals	22
Clinics	185
Clinics owned/supported for uninsured/low-income patients	18
Acute hospital admissions	140,141
Acute patient days	519,407
Emergency room visits	482,013
Inpatient surgeries	41,002
Ambulatory surgeries	107,587
Births	30,873
Patient visits to low-income clinics (owned or supported)	260,817
Employees	33,000
Affiliated physicians	2,500
Employed physicians	1,000
SelectHealth members	600,000

Source: Intermountain Healthcare (2013a).

MISSION AND PURPOSE

From Intermountain's earliest years, its mission was "excellence in the provision of healthcare services to communities in the Intermountain region." Excellent service to patients, customers, and physicians was the company's most important consideration.

VISION STATEMENT

Intermountain's formal vision statement emphasized its intent to be a model healthcare system by continually learning and providing extraordinary care in all its dimensions (Intermountain Healthcare 2013b):

- **Clinical Excellence:** We will deliver the best clinical care in a consistent, integrated way.
- **Patient Engagement:** We will provide a compassionate healing experience, and we will engage patients in decisions about their health and care.
- **Operational Effectiveness:** We will be wise and careful stewards of our resources to enable Extraordinary Care.
- **Physician Engagement:** We will create systems and processes that help our physicians best serve their patients.
- **Community Stewardship:** We are committed to serving the diverse needs of the Intermountain region and to providing generally available medical services to all residents, regardless of ability to pay.
- **Employee Engagement:** We value our employees as our most important resource.

CORE VALUES

The company's values, publicly posted and widely embraced, were as follows (Intermountain Healthcare 2013b):

- **Mutual respect:** We treat others the way we want to be treated.
- **Accountability:** We accept responsibility for our actions, attitudes, and mistakes.
- **Trust:** We act with integrity and can count on each other.
- **Excellence:** We do our best at all times and look for ways to improve.

COMPANY ETHICS

Every day, patients, health plan members, and their families came to Intermountain in need, trusting the system's providers to deliver the very best medical care and service. Intermountain's employees were committed to honoring their trust by providing excellent clinical care and superior service with the highest standards of integrity. This commitment applied to every aspect of the company's work—and was fundamental to its mission, vision, and values. Intermountain expected every one of its employees, clinicians, trustees, vendors, contractors, and volunteers to understand and follow the rules and requirements that applied to their work.

General Ethics Standards

1. We are committed to Intermountain's values of Trust, Excellence, Accountability, and Mutual Respect.

2. We perform our jobs and assignments with the highest standards of honesty and integrity. We treat each other, our patients and members, business partners, vendors and competitors fairly.

3. We know, abide by and understand the specific laws, policies and procedures that apply to our jobs and assignments, and to us as individuals.

4. We speak up with concerns about compliance and ethics issues. Specifically, we report observed and suspected violations of laws or policies, and we agree to report any requests to do things we believe may be violations. Furthermore, we cooperate with any investigation of potential violations.

5. We recognize that our daily work gives us each the opportunity to see problems in our local areas before they become apparent to others or to management. We are empowered and responsible to raise questions about potentially noncompliant or unethical practices.

6. If we have questions about a situation, we ask for help. We may talk to our supervisor or director, the facility/entity compliance coordinator, a company attorney, the Corporate Compliance Officer, or call the 24-hour Compliance Hotline at (800) 442–4845.

Source: Intermountain Healthcare (2011).

INTERMOUNTAIN'S INTEGRATED APPROACH

Intermountain's evolution into an integrated system was completed in phases. When the organization was founded in 1975, it comprised 15 hospitals. By 1985, it was a multi-hospital system that granted its facilities such a degree of autonomy that they actually competed with each other. SelectHealth (then called IHC Health Plans) had recently been created, but it existed as a satellite business and interacted little with other parts of Intermountain. Nearly all the physicians who practiced at Intermountain were independent.

◆ The first phase of integration (1985–1992) was the integration of Intermountain hospitals. The hospitals were reorganized into regions, and their governing boards followed suit. Management was consolidated and took on regional responsibilities. Intermountain hospitals began to cooperate instead of compete with each other.

◆ The second phase of integration (1992–present) was system integration. By the mid-1990s, Intermountain had all the pieces in place to make vertical integration work: hospitals, the Intermountain Medical Group of employed physicians, and SelectHealth.

BENEFITS OF HEALTH SYSTEM INTEGRATION

In the mid-1980s and early 1990s, much had been written about the need for and benefits of integrating the sometimes disparate components of hospitals and healthcare systems. From Intermountain's perspective, the internal and marketplace benefits of integration included the following:

◆ *Clinical quality.* As stated at the beginning of this case, whether through its clinical programs or by improving the treatment of certain chronic diseases, all three Intermountain divisions—Hospitals/Health Services, SelectHealth, and the Intermountain Medical Group—contributed in essential ways to the sharing of best medical practices and raising the standards of clinical excellence. For example, in treating diabetes, SelectHealth helped educate all its enrollees about the causes, dangers, and warning signs of diabetes. Members diagnosed with diabetes were contacted regularly by SelectHealth through educational materials and reminders about tests they needed to help manage their disease. At the primary care level, through the Intermountain Medical Group, Intermountain offered its Diabetes Care Management program, in which care managers worked directly with patients with diabetes to help them adhere to their care plans and access the many resources available through Intermountain. For patients with diabetes who required hospitalization, the handoff between the primary care physician and the secondary care physician and hospital team was seamless. The entire Intermountain team, from health plan to hospital, communicated and worked together to ensure the patient received the best possible care.

◆ *Service quality.* One example of the way integration helped improve service quality was via SelectHealth's Member Advocates service, which health plan members called if they needed help accessing various Intermountain services. In addition, patient billing was simplified, and programs (such as My Health) enabled patients to access both their SelectHealth information and their medical records online.

◆ *Lower costs.* In the vertically integrated Intermountain organization, costs were not reduced just through economies of scale and efficient management. The really significant cost reductions were achieved by improving the total process of medical care. By identifying and implementing best medical practices, Intermountain not only provided quality healthcare; it also achieved lasting improvements in cost structures. Moreover, those savings helped Intermountain maintain the financial strength required to provide free care to those unable to pay.

◆ *Prevention.* The incentives and resources of Intermountain's doctors, hospitals, and health plans were aligned to help people stay well.

◆ *Scope of service.* With hospitals, physician clinics, health plans, home health agencies, occupational medicine clinics, and other services, Intermountain provided a seamless continuum of care.

Over the years, healthcare leaders throughout the world called on Intermountain for technical support and education on clinical research and process management.

PATIENT FOCUS

Intermountain Healthcare declared that every person who came to Intermountain for care was unique. Its patients were individuals in the physical sense, of course, but also in terms of life stories, outlooks, and personalities. Intermountain employees recognized that the healthcare they provided needed to be carefully designed with each patient's special needs in mind. Over time, Intermountain created a culture of healing connections and developed many systems to help physicians, nurses, and other caregivers provide the most effective treatments for each patient:

◆ *Research.* Through its clinical programs and services, Intermountain made the benefits of the latest research available to clinicians. The company's board of trustees established annual goals that targeted continual improvements in healthcare quality.

- *Information systems.* Intermountain developed advanced clinical information systems that equipped caregivers with sophisticated decision-support and communication tools.

- *Support for patient health.* Intermountain established prevention, wellness, and care management programs to help patients live more satisfying lives and supported them as they followed the treatment programs prescribed by their doctors.

RELATING TO THE PHYSICIAN COMMUNITY

From the beginning, Intermountain recognized that it needed to build strong relationships with physicians. In the 1980s, Intermountain began to engage physicians more meaningfully in the organization's operations and governance. On the basis of a recommendation by a joint Intermountain–physician task force, the Intermountain Medical Group (originally called the IHC Physician Division) was established in 1994. The task force highlighted a number of important tenets:

- *Quality improvement and utilization management.* Physicians direct patient care in hospitals and are critical to their efforts to improve care processes, manage utilization, and develop clinical programs.

- *Prevention.* Physicians can do more than treat and manage disease. They can also help their patients prevent illness and help reduce or even prevent hospitalizations.

- *Security.* Managed care plans are able to direct their members to certain hospitals and physicians. In the 1990s, many physicians saw an alliance with Intermountain as a way of securing both reasonable reimbursement levels and patients.

- *Practice management.* Intermountain brings financial and administrative resources to Medical Group physicians, who are then free to focus on patient care. They also are freed of most of the administrative work associated with a solo or group practice. Furthermore, they benefit from Intermountain's investment in new, computer-based clinical information systems that help take patient care to higher levels.

- *Physician recruitment.* The Intermountain area community benefits when the Medical Group creates new physician clinics located close to the patients they serve.

RELATING TO THE PAYER COMMUNITY: INTERMOUNTAIN'S FORAY INTO HEALTH INSURANCE

Until 2006, SelectHealth was known as IHC Health Plans and was presented to the public as an aspect of the Intermountain Healthcare brand. However, research showed public confusion and misperceptions about Intermountain, so as part of Intermountain's larger rebranding, IHC Health Plans was relaunched as SelectHealth. Like its parent company, SelectHealth was organized as a nonprofit, which made it accountable to the community rather than to shareholders.

Intermountain launched its first health plan in 1984. Named Health Choice, the plan was a PPO, and the first enrollees were Intermountain's own employees. By the end of 1985, 93 companies were offering Health Choice to their employees and more than 38,000 people were covered by the plan. A second product, an HMO called IHC Care, was introduced in July 1985 and had 11,000 members by year-end. In recent years, SelectHealth offered a broad range of plans to more than 500,000 members.

In summary, SelectHealth advanced Intermountain's mission in several ways:

◆   Through SelectHealth, the entire Intermountain organization remained sensitive to the financial pressures faced by those who paid healthcare bills: employers, plan members and patients, and government. Through quality improvement and prevention, Intermountain focused on ways to keep those costs as low as possible.

◆   SelectHealth supported disease management programs that promoted health. For example, as part of Intermountain's Diabetes Care Management program, members of SelectHealth who had diabetes received reminders to take advantage of special benefits, such as diabetes counseling, free glucometers, and free clinics. SelectHealth wanted to keep its members healthy for the long term because doing so increased members' quality of life and reduced cost.

◆   SelectHealth directed a predictable flow of patients to Intermountain physicians and hospitals, which helped keep the organization and its stakeholders financially secure and able to emphasize quality improvement and prevention. Through SelectHealth, Intermountain was able to work directly with many patients and customers rather than exclusively through the mediation of third-party insurance companies.

RELATING TO THE PUBLIC AT LARGE

Since its founding, Intermountain actively engaged the community, and its family-oriented image and sponsorship were present at many and varied events, including the 2002 Olympic Games, for which the company served as official medical provider. Through the years, conventional media campaigns including print advertisements, television, radio, and billboards were widely used. In light of market research in the mid-2000s that suggested Intermountain's image as a large healthcare corporation seemingly undermined its focus on high quality and cost-effective care, the company changed its longtime name from Intermountain Health Care—widely referred to as IHC—to Intermountain Healthcare. The company's logo was also changed to reaffirm Intermountain Healthcare's mission to provide excellent care. In recent years, Intermountain began implementing social media and developed a robust presence on Facebook, Twitter, YouTube, and Foursquare.

Intermountain's most difficult and prolonged legal and public relations challenge arose in the 1990s, when some county governments determined that Intermountain hospitals should pay property tax because of the increasing business orientation of the healthcare industry in general. Intermountain ultimately survived this challenge and continued as a 501(c)(3) charitable organization on the basis of its numerous gifts to the community. Foremost among these gifts was nearly $300 million annually in charitable care to patients unable to pay.

Community Benefit Department

The vision of Intermountain's Community Benefit Department was to improve healthcare for low-income families and individuals in the community. Staff members worked with community nonprofit agencies, government entities, and healthcare providers to find ways to improve the delivery of healthcare received by uninsured, low-income patients. Partnerships, school and community clinics, collaborations, donations, and other gifts to the community made up the Community Benefit Department's wide array of projects and initiatives.

As a not-for-profit healthcare system, Intermountain annually reported its community benefits to the counties in which Intermountain facilities were located. Intermountain's Community Benefit Department helped with this reporting and also worked to improve healthcare for low-income families and individuals. Over time, improvements were made in such areas as access, delivery, funding, and the establishment of clinics.

STRATEGIC PARTNERSHIPS THAT MADE A DIFFERENCE

Over the years, Intermountain Healthcare collaborated with key organizations to bring the best of their worlds together for the benefit of the patients it served.

Huntsman–Intermountain

Intermountain Healthcare and Huntsman Cancer Institute at the University of Utah joined forces to give patients the best chance of winning the fight against cancer. Consequently, at most Intermountain hospitals, patients had access to Huntsman's outstanding research and Intermountain's renowned best-practice methods and patient care.

GE Healthcare

Intermountain partnered with GE Healthcare to create a new clinical information system based on the latest research about medical best practices. The Enterprise Clinical Information System was designed to transform the world of healthcare delivery.

FINANCING EXTRAORDINARY CARE

Caring about people required Intermountain to be careful about money. Intermountain Healthcare's mission of providing high-quality care at an affordable cost guided company leaders in making important financial decisions. Intermountain provided charity care and other community benefits because it was financially strong and prudently managed. At the same time, the company strived to keep its charges affordable.

BILLING AND COLLECTIONS ISSUES

Intermountain believed that no one should go without needed care because he/she feared the cost. In addition to providing high-quality care at affordable rates, Intermountain offered charitable assistance programs and billing policies that helped patients focus on getting well rather than worrying about how they would pay for care.

- *Charity care policy.* Through the years, Intermountain offered financial assistance on a sliding scale to families and individuals with incomes up to 500 percent of the federal poverty level.

- *Low interest rate.* For patients who needed to make payments on their bill, Intermountain's interest rate was significantly lower than typical rates for unsecured loans. Patients with a demonstrated financial need could set up a zero-interest payment plan. Patients willing and able to have their monthly payments automatically debited from their accounts qualified for a reduced interest rate.

- *Uninsured discounts.* Uninsured hospital patients who did not qualify for other assistance programs (e.g., Medicaid, CHIP) received an automatic 25 percent discount on their bills. These patients also received an additional 15 percent off their bills if full payment was made before service was provided (for a total discount of 40 percent) or an additional 5 percent off their bills if full payment was made within 30 days after service was provided (for a total discount of 30 percent).

- *Collections practices.* Intermountain did not use the courts to collect an unpaid medical bill unless there was evidence of fraud.

◆ *Widely publicized assistance policy.* Over the years, Intermountain informed patients and the community through a variety of means that charitable financial assistance was available, including signs, brochures, and counselors in facilities; information about charity care on billing statements; information about charitable assistance on the outside of billing envelopes; the Intermountain website; and information in Intermountain publications.

BUILDING NEW FACILITIES

As a not-for-profit healthcare system, Intermountain returned all money it earned to the community in the form of improved facilities, improved services, and lower charges. In Intermountain's first 20 years, it invested more than $1 billion in replacing and upgrading its facilities. It was anticipated that Intermountain would spend approximately $2.3 billion on capital improvements to this ambitious construction program between 2011 and 2016, all while keeping charges low. Intermountain Healthcare did not build new facilities to expand its presence. New facilities were intended to help the organization keep pace with the growing population and changing community needs and to serve underserved populations.

AWARDS AND RECOGNITIONS

Over much of the past decade, Intermountain was rated by IMS Health (a company that provided technology-based analytics and services for the global health community) as the number one integrated healthcare delivery system in the United States (or among the top four). US health policy experts and political leaders from across the political spectrum, including President Barack Obama and former Speaker of the House Newt Gingrich, singled out Intermountain as a model healthcare organization. Other notable recognitions were made by the following organizations:

◆ The College of Healthcare Information Management Executives and the American Hospital Association recognized Intermountain Healthcare for its leadership in information technology. The award also recognized Intermountain's extensive use of data mining—integrated with decision support in clinical information systems—to directly improve patient outcomes.

◆ The Gallup Organization chose Intermountain Healthcare as one of 27 companies worldwide to earn the Gallup Great Workplace Award for 2012. The award recognized these excellent companies for their extraordinary ability to create an engaging workplace culture.

◆ The annual Most Wired survey sponsored by *Hospitals & Health Networks*, the journal of the American Hospital Association, named Intermountain one of the nation's most technologically savvy hospital systems in 12 of the 13 years the survey was conducted.

◆ Gartner, Inc., a Connecticut-based information technology research and consulting group, ranked Intermountain's Supply Chain Organization among the best in the nation.

REGIONAL PERFORMANCE

As one of the leading healthcare providers in the Intermountain region, Intermountain Healthcare contributed to the region's performance by providing high-quality, affordable healthcare (Intermountain Healthcare 2012):

◆ Utah was lowest in the nation in terms of healthcare costs (Centers for Medicare & Medicaid Services, 1991–2009 data).

◆ Utah was best in the nation in terms of "avoidable hospital use and costs" (Commonwealth Fund, 2009 scorecard).

◆ Utah was lowest in the nation in terms of infant mortality (Commonwealth Fund, 2009 scorecard).

◆ Utah was second lowest in the nation in terms of "mortality amenable to healthcare" (Commonwealth Fund, 2009 scorecard).

◆ Three metropolitan areas in Utah—Ogden, Salt Lake, and Provo—were in the lowest fourth percentile in the United States in terms of healthcare costs (Thomson Reuters, 2009 data).

SUMMARY

Important lessons addressing key dimensions of strategic healthcare marketing are brought to light by understanding and reflecting on the story of Intermountain Healthcare. Among these lessons are the importance of mission, vision, and values in setting strategic direction and establishing organizational culture; effectively communicating an organization's development and improvement initiatives; identifying and relating to patient, physician, payer, and community stakeholders; developing strategic partnerships; and linking financial goals and plans to an organization's mission, vision, and values.

DISCUSSION QUESTIONS

1. Describe Intermountain Healthcare's attitude toward the individual patient.
2. In what ways did Intermountain engage the public at large?
3. Describe Intermountain's approach to engaging the physician community.
4. How did Intermountain relate to the insurance community?
5. Describe two or more of Intermountain's strategic alliances. How could these partnerships be marketed for maximum impact?
6. How might you describe Intermountain's approach to leadership and teamwork?
7. How did Intermountain link its financial goals to its organization-wide mission?
8. In what ways did Intermountain use market and other research to fulfill its mission?
9. What were Intermountain's most important strategic advantages? How would you market these advantages to advance the organization's mission?

REFERENCES

Intermountain Healthcare. 2013a. *Engaging All of Us in Healthcare: Intermountain Healthcare Annual Report 2012*. http://intermountainhealthcare.org/about/overview /annual-report-2012/Pages/home.html.

———. 2013b. "Mission, Vision, Values." http://intermountainhealthcare.org/about /overview/Pages/mission.aspx.

———. 2012. *Intermountain Healthcare Annual Report 2011*. http://intermountainhealthcare .org/about/overview/annualreport2011/Pages/home.html.

———. 2011. *Code of Ethics*. Created February 23; modified August 31. http://intermount ainhealthcare.org/about/overview/Documents/IntermountainCodeOfEthics.pdf.

CHAPTER 13

BUDGETING BASICS

After studying this chapter, you will be able to

➤ discuss the concept of planning and budgeting in marketing/public relations,

➤ explain return on investment for marketing projects, and

➤ create and defend a marketing budget for a project.

CASE STUDY: MONEY AND MARKETING

Christopher Echohawk wished he had paid more attention in his college healthcare finance course. His supervisor, the marketing director at Pawnee Medical Center (PMC), had given him a USB flash drive containing different reports. The director had told Christopher to look over the reports and prepare and defend the following year's budget (2015) for Pawnee Doctor Visits, a lecture series designed to educate and inform the public about various healthcare issues, for the four affiliated hospital sites of PMC. He had asked if Christopher had any questions. Christopher had replied, "No questions, I will get right on this! Thank you."

Christopher was a senior at the local university, majoring in health services management. The last class required for graduation was the internship course, which required him to complete 160 hours working in a healthcare setting. Christopher knew this internship was valuable and offered him critical experience that could parlay into a real job after graduation. Christopher liked interning in the marketing department at PMC and hoped he could join the PMC marketing staff. The people who worked in the office were smart and fun. He liked working at a medical center that employed more than 9,000 people at five different sites. And he knew he was fulfilling an important mission for the community—he was helping communicate to the public the ways in which PMC delivered excellent healthcare, and he was helping set up avenues for the public to learn more about health and wellness.

All marketing and public relations activities were discussed, implemented, and assessed with PMC's mission in mind:

> Our mission is to create and operate a comprehensive system to provide healthcare and related services, including education and research opportunities, for the benefit of the people we serve.

Christopher's internship project was to prepare for, attend, and assess Pawnee Doctor Visits. The lecture series had become popular at the four affiliated sites; each lecture had drawn about 75 to 80 attendees, and the physicians who had been involved had let the director know that their opinions about Pawnee Doctor Visits were positive. They liked speaking and visiting with the people who were interested in the subject matter.

The public learned about Pawnee Doctor Visits via word of mouth, a PMC community newsletter, and postcard mailings to residents. The postcards served as a reminder to the residents at each affiliated site to let attendees know who would be giving each lecture, what the lecture would be about, when and where the lecture would take place, and why it was being given (see Exhibit 13.1). A physician from one of the affiliated healthcare sites delivered a lecture on his or her area of expertise at one of the facilities. Twelve lectures were given annually, and speakers rotated among the four affiliated sites. Thus, each site held two to three lectures per year. Last month, Christopher attended Dr. Koda's lecture at the affiliated site in Shawnee City, located about 20 miles (a 30-minute drive) from the

---

Exhibit 13.1
Postcard for
Pawnee Doctor
Visits

LOGO of PMC HOSPITAL HERE

PMC, SHAWNEE CITY

Pawnee Medical Center, Shawnee City Pawnee Doctor Visits

WHO: Dr. William Koda, Pediatrician
WHAT: Learn About Type 2 Diabetes in Children
WHEN: Thursday, February 20, 2014, 7:00 p.m.
WHERE: Pawnee Medical Center, Shawnee City. Barook Auditorium.

Dr. Koda will be speaking about type 2 diabetes in children. Attend to learn about what symptoms to look for and how to help our children be healthy. Ask Dr. Koda questions and learn more about type 2 diabetes and our children with your neighbors.

Light refreshments served.

If you have questions, please contact Rose Hinto, Marketing, Pawnee Medical Center, by e-mail (hintor@pawneemed.com) or phone (1-800-000-0000).

---

flagship hospital, about type 2 diabetes in children. Dr. Koda identified the symptoms of the disease, discussed the need for regular exercise and good nutritional habits, and emphasized the importance of seeing a healthcare provider if one's child exhibited the symptoms. After the lecture, Christopher saw about half a dozen parents go up and talk with Dr. Koda and continue the discussion about type 2 diabetes and what they could do to help their children. These lectures mattered, and Christopher was proud to play even a small part in them.

An added benefit of Pawnee Doctor Visits for the community as well as the hospital was that some of the attendees who did not have a family pediatrician now had an opportunity to meet a local pediatrician who had privileges at PMC. Although the evidence was anecdotal, Christopher had followed up with Dr. Koda's office manager and learned that some of the attendees did make an appointment with Dr. Koda. Pawnee Doctor Visits were educating the community, but they also were a way to brand PMC positively and help connect patients to physicians.

Also anecdotal evidence of success was the positive physician feedback. The physicians who had been lecturing liked the events because they were able to discuss for an hour a topic that was of interest to them with people who were interested as well. Moreover, they reported back to the director of marketing that following the lectures they liked talking with people one-on-one about topics that mattered. The director had complimented Christopher on his efforts when he shared the positive physician feedback. "One of our goals at PMC is to develop and maintain positive relationships with our physicians."

PMC's flagship site was in a major city (population 400,000), and its affiliated hospitals were located in four other cities and towns (populations averaging 10,000 to 50,000 each) in the more rural surrounding counties. The four affiliated sites primarily focused on family care, labor and delivery, orthopedics, and general surgery. If patients from these smaller cities and more rural centers needed to see an oncologist, for example, they would travel to the flagship site for diagnosis and follow-up but receive radiation therapy or chemotherapy treatments at one of the four affiliated sites. Each was operated by PMC, each was not-for-profit, and each was a source of pride for its surrounding community. The affiliated sites were "their hospitals," and PMC marketing efforts were directed toward keeping this sense of pride and connection to the affiliated PMC sites. Hence, the popular Pawnee Doctor Visits were becoming more closely scrutinized as one way to keep the connection strong.

Christopher wanted to do a great job for the director. He returned to his cubicle in the department, put the USB flash drive into the port on his computer, and opened the files. The filenames read "Mission_of_PMC," "Department_of_Marketing_Expenses_Budget_2015_Draft," and "Budgeted_Expensed Pawnee_Doctor_Visits_2014." Christopher paused and wondered why he hadn't paid more attention in his finance course.

Planning and Budgeting in Marketing and Public Relations

While healthcare marketers do not create a medical center's budget such as PMC's annual budget and an operations plan, marketing directors are accountable for **expense** budgets for the department and all members of the marketing team are accountable for projects (e.g., Pawnee Doctor Visits). Knowledge of planning and budgeting—a degree of **financial literacy**—serves healthcare marketers as they plan, implement, and assess any marketing effort.

In the case study, Christopher was asked to plan next year's budget for a particular project—Pawnee Doctor Visits. As Gapenski (2012, 253) stated, "one could argue . . . that planning and budgeting are the most important of all finance-related tasks." In the planning process, marketers are mindful of the strategic mission of the healthcare organization in which they work. A **budget** is a statement that indicates financial administration for a set period. Take, for example, PMC. As Christopher worked on the project assigned to him, he would have been mindful of five points:

1. *Who the organization was:* What was the mission of PMC? The statement read that it was to create and operate a comprehensive system to provide healthcare and related services, including education and research opportunities, for the benefit of the people it served. The Pawnee Doctor Visits project fit well with PMC's mission, particularly given that it included educational opportunities and was directed toward the public, patients, and physicians. It educated interested parties, introduced potential patients to practitioners, helped brand PMC positively, and created an environment in which physicians were able to spend more time with people to talk about health issues.

---

expenses
costs incurred by a department's actions

financial literacy
knowledge and comprehension of financial matters

budget
a statement that indicates financial administration for a set period

2. *What the organization's goals were:* What were the future-directed tasks in the case study? The marketing director told Christopher that Pawnee Doctor Visits was an ongoing project that helped meet PMC's goals of not only educating the public but also creating and maintaining positive relationships with its physicians. Budget items for the project should have reflected both of these goals.

3. *When the organization wanted the goals accomplished:* What was the project timeline? Christopher was developing the budget for the following year.

4. *Where the organization wanted the staff to focus:* In what order were the goals prioritized? Christopher was developing a budget for the four affiliated sites. Feedback from the director may have helped Christopher determine what expenses to include in the budget. An analysis of two of the files the director gave him may have helped him as well.

5. *How the project was financially sound and workable:* In a major hospital system that had budgeted expenditures of more than $500 million—with a budget of more than $500,000 for Christopher's department (see Exhibit 13.2)—a project such as Pawnee Doctor Visits would have been merely one of many marketing efforts. Nonetheless, a project's budget needs to be financially sound and enable the marketing staff to understand what they are being asked to accomplish with what resources.

THE BUDGETING PROCESS

As Christopher developed the project budget for 2015, he would have been able to examine the budgeted amount and the expensed amount for the previous year (see Exhibit 13.3). He would have conducted a **variance** analysis—an examination of the differences between budgeted and expensed amounts and identification of what caused the differences. This analysis would have helped him provide the director with more accurate information regarding allocation of expenses for the upcoming year.

variance
the difference between two items, such as the difference between what was budgeted for a set period and what was actually expensed during that time frame

By looking at Exhibit 13.3, Christopher would have determined that PMC had spent what had been budgeted for the postcard reminders. However, more money than the amounts budgeted was spent on two items—refreshments and promotional items for events (attendees were given refrigerator magnets imprinted with hospital information and door prizes). The budget for 2014 had planned for about 50 attendees per lecture. The actual turnout had been about 75 per lecture. The variance would have been explained by the fact that 50 percent more people showed up for the events than had been expected. Hence, the expenditures reflected a 50 percent increase.

EXHIBIT 13.2

Department of
Marketing and
Public Relations_
Expenses_
Budget_2015_Draft

Account Description	Fiscal Year 2015 Proposed	Comments
Printing	$600	Stationery, business cards, office supplies
Catering	$8,000	Employee and physician events
Media and public relations	$150,000	Media buys: billboards, radio, print
Promotional	$223,000	Newsletter to public, out-sourced, agreements. Call center, outsourced. Direct-mail campaigns. Community health events. Social media projects. *Need Christopher's input here. Pawnee Doctor Visits.*
Ad development	$40,000	Agreements, consults
Web presence	$15,000	Agreements and updates
Promotional items for events	$10,000	Branding
Physician outreach	$40,000	Physician communications, physician newsletter, support for physician outreach specialist
Internal communications	$22,000	Employee forums, in-house newsletter, videos, annual report
Total	$508,600	*Draft*

The budget that Christopher returned to the director would have included a budgeted amount that accounted for growth in attendance. Because the lectures had been well received by the public and the physicians, Christopher would have increased the amount budgeted for refreshments and promotional items. He also would have considered that word of mouth about the lectures had been positive and that the newsletter that was mailed four times per year would be highlighting the lectures. The publicity associated with the article would have boosted attendance as well.

Healthcare marketers are focused on planning, budgeting, implementing, and assessing projects that will (hopefully) yield a return on investment (ROI) for the healthcare

Item	Budgeted	Expensed	Variance	
Postcards and mailing	$15,000	$15,000	—	**EXHIBIT 13.3** Budgeted_ Expensed Pawnee_ Doctor_Visits_2014
Refreshments	$1,200	$1,800	$600	
Promotional items for events	$1,200	$1,800	$600	

organization. (ROI was introduced and defined in Chapter 11.) In the case of a project such as Pawnee Doctor Visits, ROI is measured by attendance, physician response, and follow-up appointments made with physician offices. ROI is measured not only in terms of financial gain; also to be considered is the spread of positive branding, measured by the number of contacts made and the building of relationships between providers and patients as well as the public and the healthcare institution.

CHAPTER QUESTIONS

1. Explain why it is important to evaluate variances between what had been budgeted and what actually was expensed in the budget planning process.
2. Explain how ROI was measured for the Pawnee Doctor Visits project. Why was ROI not measured by a dollar amount?
3. What factors should Christopher have considered as he prepared the budget for Pawnee Doctor Visits? What else should he have considered including to make Pawnee Doctor Visits even more successful? How would he have included these factors in a budget proposal?

CHAPTER EXERCISES

1. *Christopher's budget*

   With reference to the case study, prepare the Pawnee Doctor Visits budget that you think Christopher would have sent to the director. Explain why you budgeted the items you did and how much you budgeted for the project. Remember that 12 lectures are given annually at four different sites; in 2014 the average turnout was 75 attendees per lecture.

2. *Social media and the Cancer Center*

   You are a student majoring in health services management. It is your last semester in the program, and your internship site is a hospital that would like to use social media to brand the hospital, increase public awareness on its cancer center's national ranking in *US News & World Report*'s Best Hospitals report for 2013, and elaborate on the hospital's healthcare initiatives and its leadership in providing excellent healthcare (see http://health.usnews.com/best-hospitals/rankings/cancer). You are asked to create a plan that utilizes social media to publicize and humanize the hospital's excellence.

   As you plan, examine the social media sites of other hospitals (e.g., Mayo Clinic's social media site at http://socialmedia.mayoclinic.org). Also consider who your organization is and identify its goals and how social media may be a tool that fits with its mission and might help meet those goals. Prepare an expense budget that reflects the social media tools you will use to enhance communication (e.g., consider video costs to showcase heartfelt testimonials by cancer survivors or plan an open house at the cancer center and publicize it via social media). Last, how would you evaluate your plan's success?

REFERENCE

Gapenski, L. 2012. *Healthcare Finance*, fifth edition. Chicago: Health Administration Press.

CHAPTER 14

STRATEGIC MARKETING

After studying this chapter, you will be able to

➤ discuss the concept of strategic marketing in marketing/public relations;

➤ explain the role of mission, vision, and values in marketing efforts;

➤ apply the concepts of SWOT analysis, target markets, and branding in healthcare marketing efforts; and

➤ evaluate the role of the healthcare marketer in relation to the importance of strategic marketing.

CASE STUDY: NORTHEASTERN STATE HEALTH COMMUNITY CENTERS AND OUTREACH

Sandy Krause, director of outreach and development for the six Northeastern State Health Community Centers (NEHCC), reviewed the report Tom Bartlett, sales representative from the local television station, had left with her. She had first met Tom two weeks earlier when he arrived unannounced to encourage her to purchase television advertising for NEHCC.

At first she had not been interested in television advertising for NEHCC. However, Tom showed her data that specified when people watched television and—more important to Sandy's concerns with NEHCC—data that listed which television shows were watched, the time the shows were watched, and who was watching them. Tom told Sandy that television viewing varied by family income; Tom's television company had conducted research and knew who watched what and when they watched it and the differences between television viewing behaviors by income level. This information was indeed important to Sandy and her work at NEHCC.

Sandy was glad to see the television research. It would be helpful to her as she pondered whether or not to recommend that NEHCC advertise via television as part of its outreach to communities.

NEHCC AS A PATIENT-CENTERED MEDICAL HOME

NEHCC comprised six not-for-profit healthcare community centers funded by the Bureau of Primary Health Care to deliver community and migrant healthcare needs. Primary healthcare was provided regardless of ability to pay, and the providers treated patients regardless of health insurance status (i.e., whether they had health insurance or not). The mission of NEHCC was "Empowering our patients and communities by proactively providing quality, affordable patient-centered healthcare."

NEHCC was recognized as a **patient-centered medical home (PCMH)** by the National Committee for Quality Assurance (NCQA; see www.ncqa.org). As a PCMH, the community centers were recognized as a healthcare delivery organization that ensured each patient had an ongoing relationship with a team of healthcare providers—that is, the patients saw providers they had seen before when they returned for primary healthcare (Kovner and Knickman 2011, 195). For instance, if a mother brought her son back to one of the healthcare centers for immunizations, her child was treated by the same team that had treated him earlier. Consequently, a long-term health relationship was built between provider, mother, and son if the mother and son continued coming to NEHCC. Moreover, as a PCMH, NEHCC would have sent a reminder to the mother that it was time for her son to receive the immunizations to ensure up-to-date, continuous primary care delivery. NEHCC also made certain that all communications were available in both English and Spanish.

patient-centered medical home (PCMH) a healthcare organization designed to provide comprehensive primary care for patients throughout their lives; patients have a "medical home" where healthcare providers, acting on interdisciplinary teams, provide coordinated care so that patients' information is stored at one site

As reported by NCQA (2011):

> The Patient Centered Medical Home is a health care setting that facilitates partnerships between individual patients, and their personal physicians, and when appropriate, the patient's family. Care is facilitated by registries, information technology, health information exchange and other means to assure that patients get the indicated care when and where they need and want it in a culturally and linguistically appropriate manner.

The PCMH model fit well with NEHCC's mission to deliver primary care regardless of income or insurance status and NEHCC's dedication to providing healthcare to anyone who needed it. And Sandy emphasized NEHCC's vision—to improve the health status of underserved populations—in all of her communications.

The values that underscored NEHCC were direct and simple, and every action by the healthcare teams at NEHCC endorsed and reinforced them. NEHCC's values could be summed up as "Everybody deserves good healthcare." Outreach efforts were geared toward two goals:

1. Increasing community awareness of NEHCC
2. Increasing services used at NEHCC (among both new and returning patients)

Particularly because of NEHCC's commitment to providing access to healthcare, the target markets were primarily persons with low incomes who had Medicaid or were uninsured or underinsured (i.e., they earned too much money to qualify for Medicaid but not enough to purchase comprehensive health insurance).

To that end, any efforts by Sandy and her colleagues at NEHCC should have focused on persons who may not have had full access to private physician offices, clinics, or other healthcare delivery sites that charged a set fee per visit (NEHCC charged on a sliding fee scale) or did not accept patients who could not pay for services or could not pay the copayment required by their insurance plans. Patients who may not have had full access to the aforementioned sites might have been going to the emergency department at their local hospital for primary care needs (e.g., for the flu), a costly and inefficient method of accessing care.

When Tom introduced Sandy to his company's research on television viewer status and pitched the use of television advertising, he had shown her that single mothers who earned low incomes watched Saturday morning cartoons with their children and would see an NEHCC commercial if it aired on Saturday mornings during the cartoons. Tom proposed that NEHCC's outreach efforts should target this market because these mothers were the ones who would bring their children to NEHCC for primary care if they knew about the organization and its services.

Tom also proposed that NEHCC could show the commercial in Spanish and English ten times during the Saturday morning cartoons. For each 30 seconds of commercial time NEHCC purchased, the television station would offer a 1:1 match. Hence, each commercial would average $2.50 per showing, or $25 total per Saturday. If Sandy used her own staff as the actors and used voiceovers supplied by the television station, she would incur no other costs to create or produce the commercial. Sandy knew that NEHCC received on average $111 in reimbursement from Medicaid for each Medicaid primary care visit. If the Saturday commercial spots brought in one patient, the $25 investment would return $86 to NEHCC.

Sandy edited the excerpted section from NEHCC's strategic marketing plan to include outreach commercials. (See Exhibit 14.1; Sandy's edits are italicized.) She considered the following questions: Would such an action help meet the objective of advertising outreach? The goal of increasing community awareness? Did it fit with NEHCC's mission, vision, and values? Did it fit as part of a marketing strategy that would enable NEHCC to concentrate its limited resources on its greatest opportunities, increase sales, attain its goals, and achieve a sustainable competitive advantage (Baker 2008, 3)? Moreover, she remained aware of the importance that any strategic success would be dependent on NEHCC's outreach initiatives—its relationships with referring physicians, clinics, and hospitals as well as ongoing relationships with patients and the public.

Strategic Healthcare Marketing and the Importance of Mission, Vision, and Values

strategic planning
design of a plan to achieve agreed-upon goals

As discussed in Chapter 3, **strategic planning** is the design of a plan to achieve agreed-upon goals. NEHCC had established two overarching goals:

1. Increasing community awareness of NEHCC

2. Increasing services used at NEHCC (among both new and returning patients)

As the director of outreach and development, part of Sandy's job was to reach out to referring physicians, clinics and hospitals, potential patients, and the public so that people were made aware of NEHCC's services. This outreach required marketing efforts. To ensure that appropriate efforts are implemented, persons in positions such as Sandy's must possess a clear understanding of what their healthcare organization is and know the environment in which the organization exists. To build this understanding, some organizations hold formal strategic planning retreats; others are more informal and hold strategic planning meetings. The main point is that the organization's administrators, board members, and clinical managers strategize about how to meet agreed-upon goals. Moreover, any agreed-upon goals, objectives, and actions should fit with the organization's mission (who it is), vision (where it wants to be), and values (how it wants to go about achieving its mission and vision).

EXHIBIT **14.1**
Advertising
Section—Excerpt
from NEHCC's
Strategic
Marketing Plan

Goal 1: Increase community awareness of NEHCC

Objective 3: Maximize advertising outreach efforts

Action	Target Date	Frequency	Person Responsible	Comments
Radio—research commercial with radio stations	September 15	Biweekly	Sandy	Identify best value stations (in progress; have contacted a few stations).
Spanish phone-book listing	Done	Yearly	Sandy	$200 annual fee. Non-Spanish listing too expensive.
Research billboards	October 15	??	Sandy	More likely to be cost-effective in rural areas. May donate?
Research television	*September 15*	*Biweekly*	*Sandy*	*$2.50 per 30-second commercial if run 10x; bilingual commercials. Total investment $20.50 per Saturday.*

Market research to assess the environment also contributes significantly to the success of strategic initiatives. Research conducted by an organization may include patient satisfaction surveys; patients are asked questions regarding how they heard about the healthcare site and regarding their experiences at the site. An organization also may benefit from research conducted by outside organizations. In the case study, Tom shared with Sandy the research conducted by the television station to identify television-viewing behavior.

Large hospitals may outsource some of their marketing research needs. For instance, one hospital was interested in learning if a cardiovascular center would add value to the region and be profitable for the hospital. The hospital hired a firm from another state to study the demographics (i.e., age, income level, and health status of area residents) and competition (i.e., what cardiovascular services other healthcare organizations within a 50-mile, 100-mile, and 150-mile radius offered) in the area. Whether the organization is conducting its own research or using research provided by an objective, outside firm, the fact remains that market research helps clarify the goals of the organization, identify target markets, and direct branding efforts.

SWOT Analysis, Target Markets, Branding, and Promotion Methods

SWOT analysis

a tool used to iden-
tify an organization's
internal strengths and
weaknesses as well as
an organization's exter-
nal opportunities and
threats

A **SWOT analysis** (strengths, weaknesses, opportunities, and threats) is one tool that may be used to identify an organization's internal strengths and weaknesses as well as an organization's external opportunities and threats. SWOT analyses are subjective, a result of stakeholders' opinions. *Stakeholders* are individuals, groups, and entities that have an interest in an organization's success. With reference to NEHCC, stakeholders would have included the organization's executive director, board of directors, clinical managers, and administrative staff (including Sandy). Because NEHCC was funded by the Bureau of Primary Health Care as community and migrant health centers, 51 percent of the board members were clinic users. Hence, patients were represented as well. (For more information about health centers and a description of Health Center Program fundamentals, see http://bphc.hrsa.gov.)

Often a SWOT survey is distributed to stakeholders prior to the strategic planning retreat or meeting, and the results are distributed to attendees and discussed at the retreat/meeting. On the basis of this discussion, the organization establishes goals to work toward. For an example, consider the SWOT analysis conducted by NEHCC prior to its strategic planning retreat (see Exhibit 14.2).

From the SWOT analysis, the stakeholders who attended the NEHCC strategic planning retreat determined that an opportunity for NEHCC was to focus on Medicaid patients (new and returning). The target market they identified, therefore, was Medicaid recipients. The number of new patients was expected to increase after Medicaid coverage was expanded, and the state in which NEHCC was located had indicated it would accept the expanded Medicaid provision, which was scheduled to take effect in 2014 per the Affordable Care Act (Medicaid.gov 2013). (Remember that in 2012 the US Supreme Court ruled that states may or may not accept Medicaid expansion; see www.supremecourt.gov/opinions/11pdf/11-393c3a2.pdf.)

Also, the attendees determined that the image of NEHCC—its branding—should be improved. Comments such as "they are just free clinics" needed to be addressed and the public be made aware that NEHCC was for all patients who needed care, regardless of racial or ethnic origin. The American Marketing Association (2013) defines *brand* as "a name, term, design, symbol, or any other feature that identifies one seller's good or service as distinct from those of other sellers." The branding of service products involves consumers as co-creators of the branding image (Anker et al. 2011). Hence, in the case study, the service was primary healthcare, the consumers were the patients of NEHCC, and the patients and the sites were the co-creators of the "brand experience and brand benefit" (Anker et al. 2011, 34). To effectively brand NEHCC, both NEHCC and the patients would have had to embrace the idea that the patient experience at NEHCC resulted in quality healthcare. NEHCC had to become associated with positive, desirable images of health providers who offered healthcare for everyone. The best way to bring about this branding was strategic marketing, or in Sandy's case, the success specifically would have

Strengths	Weaknesses	**EXHIBIT 14.2**

EXHIBIT 14.2
NEHCC's SWOT
Analysis

Strengths	Weaknesses
• Committed employees dedicated to NEHCC	• Community image (perception of NEHCC as "just a free clinic" and "serving Hispanics only")
• Patient satisfaction is high	• Always in need of more funding
• Patients are represented on board	• Retention of quality staff
• Spanish and English speaking	• Competitive wages gap
• Friendly and caring staff	• Write-off $$$ in accounts receivable
• Has facility to accommodate more patients	
• Clinics are known to communities	
• Affordable/high-quality primary care	
• Professional development for staff provided	
• Good EMR system; good IT support	
• Accredited as PCMH	
• Six locations in region of the state	

Opportunities	Threats
• Increase in Medicaid-reimbursable clients because of Medicaid expansion (2014)	• Other healthcare sites potentially competing for patients who can pay (Medicaid)
• Recession economy increases number of patients who need NEHCC	• Provider turnover
• Federal grant due—align with NEHCC's mission	• Other healthcare sites better at marketing (getting the word out)

been dependent on NEHCC's outreach initiatives—its relationships with referring physicians, clinics, and hospitals as well as ongoing relationships with patients and the public.

HEALTHCARE MARKETERS AND STRATEGIC MARKETING EFFORTS

As healthcare marketers consider how best to design, implement, and assess marketing efforts, they are mindful of their organization's mission, vision, and values; are schooled in research findings conducted (or contracted) by the organization; and understand the organization's prioritized goals. Simply put, for any marketing effort, questions such as the following could be addressed:

1. Does this marketing effort fit with the organization's mission?

2. Will it help the organization achieve its vision?

3.   Is it consistent with the organization's values?

4.   Does it address the target market identified?

5.   Does it say what the marketing team wants it to say to physicians, patients, and the public?

6.   How would the marketing team measure its success?

For example, consider Sandy's deliberation about the television commercials for NEHCC. The commercials on Saturday mornings might have been one way to accomplish the following:

◆   Increase awareness by promoting NEHCC to a particular target market (single mothers on Medicaid who have young children)

◆   Brand NEHCC as the healthcare clinic that delivers quality healthcare for everyone

The commercials would not have been the only way to meet NEHCC's goal to increase community awareness. They would have been just one part of a marketing plan and were presented in the case study to illustrate the process healthcare marketers follow as they examine each step they plan to take to meet an identified organizational goal. One way to measure the success of an outreach effort such as the commercials would be to ask patients how they heard about the organization when they come in for an appointment. Such assessment enables healthcare marketers to determine whether or to what degree marketing efforts were successful.

CHAPTER QUESTIONS

1.   Other than the television commercials, identify another way NEHCC could have met its goal to increase community awareness. How could NEHCC have reached its target market of single mothers with young children other than via television?

2.   Explain how your answer to question #1 fits with the mission of NEHCC. How would your idea have helped achieve NEHCC's vision? Is it consistent with NEHCC's values? Does it communicate what NEHCC wanted to communicate to physicians, patients, and the public?

3.   How would you measure the success of your idea?

CHAPTER EXERCISES

1. *Assessing strategic marketing efforts*

   Ultimately, Sandy decided to implement the commercials. The transcript for the commercials follows. As you read it, consider the first six questions marketers consider as they decide whether or not to implement a marketing effort:

   a. Does this marketing effort fit with the organization's mission?
   b. Will it help the organization achieve its vision?
   c. Is it consistent with the organization's values?
   d. Does it address the target market identified?
   e. Does it say what the marketing team wants it to say to physicians, patients, and the public?
   f. How would the marketing team measure its success?

   Transcript: 30-second commercial

   (The opening statement is spoken by Sandy's eight-year old son; the visual is the boy, who is looking at the camera. NEHCC's phone number is displayed on the screen. The boy looks at the camera and says:)

   > *Everybody deserves good healthcare.*

   (A woman's voiceover follows; the visual is a family entering the clinic, and then individuals are seen speaking with healthcare providers in a friendly one-on-one atmosphere:)

   > *NEHCC has been a blessing for our family. Is a not-for-profit, federally funded community healthcare organization. It has Board Certified, caring physicians who provide care for anything from routine visits to unexpected sore throats. NEHCC's fees are based on income and family size. It accepts new Medicaid and Medicare patients. NEHCC also helps its patients save on prescriptions.*

   (A man's voiceover follows; the visual is NEHCC's logo, which shows NEHCC and the statements "Healthcare for everyone" and "Se habla español":)

   > *NEHCC, in . . .* (He lists the six locations where NEHCC is located and concludes by saying:) *NEHCC, healthcare for everyone.*

   Measuring success

   The commercials cost $25 every other week for a period of 12 months ($650 total). A survey asking "How did you hear about the community clinic?" was given to patients who came in for an appointment. The number of patients who reported that they had heard about NEHCC via the commercials was counted over the 12-month period as one measure to assess the impact of the outreach effort. If four new Medicaid patients per month reported that they had heard about NEHCC via the commercials and that they (the mothers) as well as two of their children sought healthcare at least once during the year, at least 144 patient visits resulted. At an average of $111 per visit, Sandy determined that NEHCC brought in $15,984 on a $650 investment. Moreover, given that NEHCC had the capacity to see new patients, these earnings were additional revenue. Consider question #6 from the list of questions that marketers consider as they decide whether to implement a marketing effort. Do you think the commercials were a success? Explain your answer.

2. *Preparing your own personal SWOT analysis*

    In strategic planning, stakeholders may brainstorm or be surveyed regarding their thoughts on the organization's strengths and weaknesses and the opportunities and threats the organization may respond to. This exercise is designed to get you to think about your own strengths and weaknesses as well as opportunities and threats you should be aware of. Answer the following questions:

    ### Strengths

    a. Write down at least five things you are good at.
    b. Write down at least five things you like to do (some may be a repeat of your answers to question #1).
    c. Write down three things other people say you are good at.

    ### Weaknesses

    a. Write down at least five things you feel you do not do well or could improve on.
    b. Write down at least five things you do but don't enjoy doing.
    c. Write down three things other people say you should improve on.

    ### Opportunities

    a. Write down at least three things going on "out there" (i.e., in the environment) that you could take advantage of.
    b. Write down at least two things others say you could take advantage of out there.

c. What is something in the environment that could help you achieve your goals?

Threats

a. Write down at least two things out there that could negatively affect your ability to attain your goals.
b. Write down at least two things out there that others worry could negatively affect your ability to attain your goals.
c. What is something in the environment that could stop you from doing what you do best?

Analysis

After your answer these questions, pair your strengths with your opportunities, your weaknesses with your opportunities, your threats with your strengths, and your weaknesses with your threats in a table like the following. Think about how you could match your strengths with your opportunities to achieve your goals while remaining mindful of your weaknesses. The following example may help guide you through the exercise.

	Strengths	**Weaknesses**
Opportunities	I'm good at social media. The local community center is looking for someone to help with its Facebook page. I could volunteer, offer service leadership, and add to my resume.	I'm disorganized. How can I work on time management so that I can volunteer at the community center and help with its Facebook page? I could work on my time management skills with the aid of time management aids I can find on the Web.
Threats	A threat is the economy—I have to work while I go to school full time. That's why I'm disorganized. I don't have time to get organized. Perhaps I could work on time management so that I can do all three—work, go to school, and volunteer.	I'm disorganized. How could I manage time effectively to do all three?

REFERENCES

American Marketing Association. 2013. "AMA Dictionary." www.marketingpower.com/ _layouts/Dictionary.aspx?dLetter=B.

Anker, T. B., P. Sandoe, T. Kamin, and K. Kappel. 2011. "Health Branding Ethics." *Journal of Business Ethics* 104: 33–45.

Baker, M. 2008. *The Strategic Marketing Plan Audit*. Devon, UK: Cambridge Strategy Publications.

Kovner, A., and J. Knickman. 2011. *Health Care Delivery in the United States*, tenth edition. New York: Springer Publishing Company.

Medicaid.gov. 2013. "Affordable Care Act." www.medicaid.gov/AffordableCareAct /Affordable-Care-Act.html.

National Committee for Quality Assurance (NCQA). 2011. "Patient-Centered Medical Home." www.ncqa.org/tabid/631/default.aspx.

CHAPTER 15

THE MARKETING PLAN

After studying this chapter, you will be able to

➤ identify the components of a marketing plan,

➤ create and defend a marketing plan,

➤ explain ethical issues related to healthcare marketing plans, and

➤ evaluate the role of the healthcare marketer as the plan leader from inception to assessment.

CASE STUDY: THE MARKETING PLAN AT RIVERS AND THE ROBOT

Marketing and public affairs director Belinda Sheldon and media specialist Rick Stallings were the entire office staff for marketing and public affairs at Rivers Medical. Rick was staying late in the office because Belinda had been called to attend an impromptu strategy meeting that afternoon by the hospital's executive director. Rick knew that something was about to happen that would require him and Belinda to work quickly and expertly. He called his wife and told her to go ahead and have dinner without him. He'd be home later.

Rivers Medical was a not-for-profit hospital with 237 licensed beds, more than 1,300 employees, and a physician medical staff of about 200. It served the local city and the rural surrounding towns in the rolling hills area of Tennessee. Its mission read:

> Rivers Hospital provides compassionate, quality healthcare services needed by the people of Tennessee in collaboration with other providers and community resources.

Its vision read:

> Rivers is a comprehensive regional referral center committed to providing the finest in competent, courteous, and compassionate care.

Its values read:

> These beliefs and values are the foundation of our mission and vision:
>
> Compassion—We care for others as if they are members of our own family.
>
> Dignity—We treat every person with respect.
>
> Excellence—We continually improve our services to ensure the highest quality of care.
>
> Education—We maintain a commitment to growth and learning.
>
> Accountability—We use resources wisely to ensure that services are consistently provided at appropriate cost.
>
> Collaboration—We work with others to improve the health status of the community.

Belinda entered the boardroom and acknowledged each person as he or she entered. The Rivers strategic planning team was for the most part a collegial group that worked well together and liked working together. It was a good thing to work in an environment that encouraged input and lively discussion from all areas of the hospital, both clinical and administrative. Belinda and Rick attributed this positive culture to the executive director,

Patrick Habeeb, who led the hospital with patients, physicians, the public, and payers in mind. He was known for asking purposeful questions—questions that made others think about the mission, vision, and values of Rivers. He was kind and polite, and even though he was busy, he made others feel as though he had all the time in the world for them.

Belinda nodded to the nursing director, who was followed by the medical director and whom Belinda called the C-suite—the chief financial officer (CFO), chief information officer (CIO), chief operations officer (COO), and Mr. Habeeb. Two OB/GYN surgeons accompanied Mr. Habeeb. Belinda expected the meeting to be short, as was customary when Mr. Habeeb was in charge. He was simple and direct and encouraged the rest of the strategy team to offer suggestions and formulate the plan.

The nearest hospital to Rivers, Memorial Hospital, was a 25-minute drive away. It had acquired the da Vinci robot three years earlier, primarily for OB/GYN surgery (see www. davincisurgery.com). At that time, Rivers had considered purchasing the robot. However, given that the Rivers physicians did not seem interested in the robot and given the population of the city and the surrounding towns, the Rivers strategy team had determined that there would not be enough surgeon/patient demand to utilize the robotic services profitably.

The CFO had reported that the cost of the robot would have been $1.5 million, with another $140,000 budgeted for the annual service contract. Rivers also had anticipated spending about $1,500 per year for replacement parts. Training would have involved the surgeons, the operating room nurses and staff, robotics program managers, and hospital administrators. The CFO had determined that the robot would need to perform about eight surgeries per week to be profitable. Belinda had reported that marketing research (an outsourced phone survey of city residents) had indicated positive interest in the da Vinci robot and its potential for less invasive surgery. Marketing efforts would have been directed at television, radio, billboards, websites, and community events. Success would have been measured by the number of calls directed to Rivers' call center (to track interest in robotic surgery), physicians' responses, and the actual number of surgeries performed (with a goal of more than eight per week). A marketing budget of $40,000 to promote the da Vinci robot had been proposed. The end decision was that the team could not recommend the purchase at that time, particularly in light of Memorial's decision to purchase it.

However, within the last six months, the physicians who primarily had used the da Vinci robot left Memorial to practice on the West Coast. Hence, the da Vinci robot was not being used productively because the other surgeons at Memorial were not interested in learning how to use it; they were satisfied with laparoscopic surgery because it was minimally invasive as well. As a result, Memorial stopped leasing the surgical robot.

Mr. Habeeb stated that three OB/GYN surgeons and two urologists at Rivers had let it be known that they would like Rivers to purchase a da Vinci robot. The two surgeons in attendance at the meeting spoke of the robot's benefits and how they now supported and encouraged Rivers to purchase it. The da Vinci robot allowed for minimally invasive surgery, causing less pain for the patient and less scarring than conventional surgery caused. The board of directors at Rivers had decided to take advantage of this opportunity and had approved the purchase. The CFO reported that the costs had increased slightly since their first assessment three years prior. The purchase price was $1.7 million, with a service contract of $150,000 per year. Rivers also could anticipate spending about $1,500 per year for replacement parts. Moreover, the CFO reported that the robot would still need to perform about eight surgeries per week to be profitable. The meeting had been called that afternoon to get everyone started; they needed to start doing what they needed to do to prepare for the robot's arrival, which was scheduled for delivery within the next month.

Mr. Habeeb adjourned the meeting, and Belinda rose to leave; she and Rick had much to do to implement their original marketing plan. But Mr. Habeeb asked her to remain behind. After the room emptied, he informed her that he knew her budget had been committed to other hospital marketing efforts and Rivers just didn't have the money to support her originally proposed $40,000 plan. "We do not want to take away from your other projects. I'll need you to work within a $2,200 budget, Belinda. I know we usually commit more resources, but we just cannot at this time."

Belinda joined Rick in the office and told him what Mr. Habeeb had said. "We have to write a whole new plan. Want to order a pizza? We have some brainstorming to do." Rick replied, "Pizza is already on its way. I had a feeling we would have some work to do."

MARKETING PLANS

marketing plan
a document that demonstrates how the healthcare organization will implement the already established marketing strategy

Marketing plans demonstrate how the healthcare organization will implement the already established marketing strategy. The following is a summary of the components of a marketing plan (Oetjen and Oetjen 2006, 50–56):

1. *Executive summary:* This part of the plan explains what the **situational analysis** showed, what the objectives are for the project, and how those objectives will be met. The executive summary is an overview of the plan because it incorporates factors from the next components discussed in this list (items 2 through 6).

situational analysis
an analysis (e.g., a SWOT analysis) of what is happening in an organization's external and internal environments

2. *Situational analysis:* This component refers to an analysis that utilizes tools to assess what is happening in the external and internal environments. A competitive analysis and a SWOT analysis (a subjective categorization of the healthcare organization's internal strengths and weaknesses and external opportunities and threats; see Chapter 14) may yield information for the situational analysis. In a *competitive analysis*, the strategy team assesses the healthcare organization's competitors. In the case study, Memorial was the nearest competitor with regard to use of the da Vinci robot. Its decision to stop using the robot created an opportunity for Rivers. A SWOT analysis

would have enabled the planning team to consider what is important to the hospital regarding patients, physicians, and the public.

A situational analysis may be viewed in a two-by-two matrix (Oetjen and Oetjen 2006, 51). In the case study, the marketing plan situational analysis might have looked something like the matrix in Exhibit 15.1.

3. *Market research:* Whether outsourced or conducted in-house, **market research** refers to efforts to discover and identify the needs of patients, physicians, and the public. From analysis of earlier marketing research—the outsourced phone survey mentioned in the case study had identified public interest in the da Vinci robot—and a review of the population demographics and competition, it had been determined that one of the hospitals could effectively utilize the robot, but the community population size could not support profitable utilization of the robot at both hospitals.

4. *Market strategy:* This section of the plan refers to the target market and what the organization wants to convey so that it meets the target market's needs. In the case study, primary utilization of the robot at Rivers was to be twofold—for OB/GYN and urology—because the physicians who had expressed interest in robotic surgery were from these specialties. The target market, therefore, would have been families; if Belinda and Rick succeeded at communicating their message to mothers and their families about the da Vinci robot and OB/GYN and urological procedures, they would have educated the consumer, potential patients, the public, and payers and made them aware of—and

market research
efforts to discover and identify the needs of patients, physicians, and the public; may be outsourced or conducted in-house

Exhibit 15.1
Marketing Plan Situational Analysis, Rivers Medical

Strengths	Opportunities
What does Rivers do well?	What are opportunities for Rivers?
Positive reputation; brand recognition	Need for robotic surgery option in community
100% of hospital physicians are board certified	Physicians at Memorial are not interested in robotic surgery; physicians at Rivers are interested

Weaknesses	Threats
Physicians and staff are not trained to use robot	Public is aware of Memorial's rejection of robot, which *may* have made the public question robotic surgery
Budget shortages	

market strategy

the section of the marketing plan that identifies the target market and what the organization wants to convey so that it reaches the target market effectively and meets the target market's needs

(hopefully) incited interest in—the da Vinci robot services to be offered at Rivers. Also part of **market strategy** is determining how best to reach the target market within the budget guidelines and whether the strategy is a good fit with the organization's mission, vision, and values. Finally, return on investment (ROI) needs to be identified (ROI was introduced and defined in Chapter 11). For some marketing projects, ROI might be measured in terms of the number of clicks people made on the organization's website (e.g., how many people clicked a link to watch a video of patient testimonials) or the increase in the number of patients who made an appointment with a physician.

5.   *Monitoring the plan:* Monitoring involves following up with and paying attention to marketing efforts throughout the planning and implementation processes (plan the work; work the plan). Plans may be monitored by noting participation by target market, measuring patient satisfaction or dissatisfaction, and making certain that the marketing campaign is on time and on schedule.

6.   *Ethics:* The American Marketing Association's (AMA) Statement of Ethics is clear regarding the importance of truth in advertising, promotion, and publicity. According to the AMA (2013), marketers must not do harm; must ensure that the truth is told and deception is avoided; and must act with honesty, integrity, fairness, and respect. It is the responsibility of the people involved at any stage of the marketing plan—planning, initiating the plan, and/or assessing the plan—to follow these ethical guidelines. Misrepresentation of any aspect of the da Vinci robot would have been at odds with the values of Rivers and a violation of professional responsibility.

EPILOGUE: "NAME OUR ROBOT OR DRAW OUR ROBOT" CAMPAIGN

Consider the case study and the charge to develop a marketing plan within a $2,200 budget, particularly in light of the fact that the original budget was $40,000. Belinda and Rick devised the following four-pronged strategy. Three components were to be immediately initiated and occur over a one-month period; the fourth was to begin three months later.

1.   Rick maintained the social media outlets for the hospital; he created, at no cost but his time, frequently asked questions (FAQs) about the da Vinci robot and included a link to them on the main page of the hospital's "Medical Minutes" blog. He also included the call center's number so that people could call and ask more about the robot. He measured the success of this initiative

by the number of times people clicked the link to access the list of FAQs and the number of calls made to the call center about the robot. (The call center was already budgeted under operations. The call center staff members noted what each call was about and whether or not the calls resulted in physician referrals. It was not paid for with the marketing budget but was one avenue for Rick and Belinda to publicize the da Vinci robot.) Rick also posted a picture of the robot on the hospital's Facebook page and tweeted (via Twitter) throughout the robot's travel to the hospital.

2. Belinda designed the "Name Our Robot or Draw Our Robot" campaign. She worked with every school in the city where Rivers was located. Spending $300 for the graphics, she designed a colorful flyer for the campaign. It featured a picture of the robot with "Hi, my name is _____" typed on its monitor screen and read as follows:

NAME OUR ROBOT OR DRAW OUR ROBOT

Name our robot for a chance to win $500.

The da Vinci robot is like a doctor's best friend. Our robot helps make surgery easier for patients. They have smaller scars, they don't feel as much pain, they get better faster, and best of all, they get to go home sooner.

Fill out the form on the back and give it to your teacher. If we choose the name you picked for our robot, you will receive $500 and your class will receive $500.

Draw our robot for a chance to win $100.

Draw our robot, just as you see it here or as a fun cartoon character. If we choose your drawing, you will receive $100 and your class will receive $100. We will choose one winner from each of three student categories: K–3, 4–6, and 7–12.

Community Open House.

Meet our da Vinci robot!
Friday, September 6, 2013, 6 p.m.
Rivers Medical Plaza
231 Rivers Medical Drive

All drawings will be on display, and winners will be announced.

Note: The flyers were hand-delivered to each school, and the schools gave the flyers to the teachers to distribute to the students to take home. Success was measured by the number of students who entered the contests.

3. Belinda and Rick held a community open house to unveil the new name and acknowledge the winners and their teachers. Each of the three high schools in the city had competitive robotics teams that had been the pride of the city for some time. One team had won the state robotics championship in recent history, and the other school teams were determined to do well in future robotics competitions. Rick invited the three teams to come to the community open house and display their robotics projects during the evening. All three teams accepted the invitation. Rick posted information about the community open house on the hospital's website and Facebook page, and Belinda included the same information on the "Name Our Robot or Draw Our Robot" flyer. Success was measured by attendance. Belinda arranged for refreshments at the open house at a cost of $300, and the da Vinci robot was in attendance as well so that the public could see the technology up close and in a friendly environment.

4. Three months later, Belinda and Rick filmed videos of patient testimonials and posted the videos on the hospital's website. Success was measured by the number of clicks on the video link and physicians' responses to the videos.

RETURN ON INVESTMENT

In their book *Marketing Matters*, Richard Thomas and Michael Calhoun (2007, 138) propose that the "best measures in healthcare are softer measures like goodwill, awareness, and public relations coverage." In the case study, readers' responses to social media, attendance at the open house, and receipt of contest entries were ways to assess the degree of goodwill, awareness, and public relations coverage Rivers had attained.

Adding an incentive for teachers (i.e., the potential to win money for their classes) was another way to ensure that the flyers went home with the students, and it also created goodwill between the schools and the local hospital. ROI included the following:

♦   The link to the FAQs was clicked 100 times in the first week.

♦   The call center received 50 calls about the robot in the first two weeks.

♦   The number of Facebook likes totaled 350 within the first week.

These numbers indicated a degree of public interest in and awareness of the da Vinci robot at Rivers. Entries in the "Name Our Robot or Draw Our Robot" campaign exceeded 1,000. More than 500 people attended the open house, and comments were made about the goodwill Rivers had generated by supporting the high school robotics teams. The cost of the campaign was $2,200.

Belinda reported that the winning name was "Wanda, because the robot had magic wands for hands." Physicians' responses were overwhelmingly positive, and within three months, utilization of the da Vinci robot at Rivers exceeded eight per week and reached capacity within six months.

HEALTHCARE MARKETERS AS STRATEGIC THINKERS AND CREATIVE PLANNERS

A strong case can be made for the role of healthcare marketers and applying marketing principles, techniques, and practices exemplified by the "Name Our Robot or Draw Our Robot" campaign to inform the public, particularly families, about Rivers Medical's acquisition of the da Vinci robot. The campaign fit nicely with the mission, vision, and values of Rivers, and the focus on school children (kindergarten through high school) created a unique opportunity for the public to embrace the robot as its robot and engendered a sense of community pride. Healthcare marketing really is more than selling to the public. Healthcare marketers educate and inform patients and the public and work with physicians and payers to greatly enhance the health and well-being of the public—individuals, communities, and society.

CHAPTER QUESTIONS

1. Prepare the $2,200 budget that Belinda and Rick implemented for the da Vinci robot campaign. Refer to Chapter 13 for the basics of budgeting.
2. Belinda's and Rick's campaign was indeed creative, given their reduced budget. Name two other ways they might have reached their target market if their funding had not been reduced.
3. After physicians perform surgeries via the da Vinci robot, Belinda and Rick could film videos of patient testimonials and could post the videos on the hospital's website. What other social media would you have included in their marketing plan regarding the da Vinci robot?

CHAPTER EXERCISES

1. *The da Vinci robot*

   Go to the website that markets the da Vinci robot (www.davincisurgery.com). Assess the site. What social media tools are used to define, describe, and promote the robot?

Overall, is the site effective? Does it offer information about the robot and why it is a good idea for surgery? Is it easy for users to navigate and comprehend the information given? What other social media tools could be used to educate the public about this technology?

2. *Executive summary*

Refer to the case study in this chapter. You have the information you need to write a two-page (typed, 12-point font, double-spaced) executive summary to Mr. Habeeb, the executive director. Write the executive summary. As you write it, consider why value is added by including each part elaborated on in this chapter in the plan (i.e., situational analysis, market research, and market strategy that identifies target markets). Also explain why value is added by focusing on physicians, patients, and the public when developing the plan. Finally, evaluate Belinda's and Rick's marketing campaign. Do you think their efforts succeeded at educating the public about Rivers Medical's acquisition of the robot? About the benefits of robotic surgery? Were you surprised to learn that the surgeons' responses to the plan were positive? That utilization was at capacity within six months of the event?

REFERENCES

American Marketing Association (AMA). 2013. "Statement of Ethics: Ethical Norms and Values for Marketers." www.marketingpower.com/AboutAMA/Pages/Statement%20of%20Ethics.aspx.

Oetjen, R., and D. Oetjen. 2006. *Medical Practice Management Body of Knowledge Review: Planning and Marketing, Volume 7*. Englewood, CO: MGMA.

Thomas, R. K., and M. Calhoun. 2007. *Marketing Matters*. Chicago: Health Administration Press.

GLOSSARY

adjourning: the final stage of teamwork; members review outcomes and disengage from the team

ambulatory care: healthcare services that do not require an overnight stay in a hospital; also called *outpatient care*

attitudes: individuals' internal states, which affect a team's ability to work together

authority: the ability of someone in a position of power to direct others to take some action

autonomy: respectful behavior toward other persons and mindfulness of the importance of truth and confidentiality

behaviors: the application of skills, actions, and abilities necessary to accomplish the work

beneficence: ensuring that one's behaviors benefit others and do no harm

board certification: an official status reflecting mastery of a specialty, granted by professional agencies and organizations to physicians who pass an advanced examination; maintained by yearly completion and documentation of continuing medical education

brand management: controlling and influencing the relationship between an organization's customers and its readily identifiable and publicly recognized products or services

brand touch point *or* **brand contact point:** any contact or interaction that reinforces an organization's brand or marketing message

branding: establishing positive associations with an organization in the minds of customers (In healthcare, customers are patients, physicians, and the public.)

budget: a statement that indicates financial administration for a set period

charisma: a quality of inspiring role models that comes from having strong, visible values and an ability to attract and maintain loyalty

communication channel: the method or medium through which a message or information is communicated

community benefits: activities, programs, and healthcare provided to promote and enhance quality of life among the community at large

confidence: recognition of one's own abilities and skills; the state of being consciously competent

conflict: a state of disharmony or lack of agreement between at least two parties over ideas, beliefs, or practices

consciously competent: knowing what works, with whom it works, and why it works

controlling: monitoring and evaluating the plan, the tasks, and completion of the tasks and the project

cost as a proxy for quality: the use of cost as an indicator of a product's quality when true information regarding quality is absent; the belief that the more expensive a product is, the higher its quality

credentialing: an in-depth background, education, and practice investigation performed by a hospital to determine whether a physician is qualified to receive medical staff privileges

"culturization": learning and adopting the activity and behavior deemed appropriate or required of a specific group or profession

customer: one who purchases a commodity or service

determination: initiative, persistence, and drive; staying focused and staying the course

directing: motivating, influencing, and ensuring effective and timely implementation and completion of tasks; communicating goals, deadlines, and desired outcomes

distribution avenues: channels through which information, a product, or a service is communicated or made available to target markets

dysfunctional conflict: conflict that may contribute to a decline in work performance

electronic health record (EHR): an electronic version of a patient's medical record

expenses: costs incurred by a department's actions

fee-for-service: a retrospective reimbursement system in which providers create a comprehensive list of services they provided to a patient and the materials, supplies, and facilities they used to provide those services and then bill the patient's insurer (or the patient, if he/she is self-pay) for each item on the list

fidelity: loyalty and faithfulness to one's professional duty

financial literacy: knowledge and comprehension of financial matters

forming: the first stage of teamwork; members are given their charge and learn the purpose of the team

functional conflict: conflict that may contribute to positive work performance

graduate medical education (GME): the years of internships, residencies, and additional training and specialization following graduation from medical school

health literacy: the degree to which one has and understands health information essential to making informed health decisions

health maintenance organization (HMO): a managed care delivery system that merges the provision of care and the reimbursement function of health insurance

health promotion: activities designed to influence individual behaviors that affect personal health

healthcare customers: patients, physicians, the public, and payers

healthcare ethics: moral standards of clinical and administrative conduct that affect healthcare stakeholders

healthcare marketing: a fine-tuned art and science that creates, communicates, and delivers offerings that have value for healthcare stakeholders, including patients, physicians, the public, and payers

healthscape: the service areas, waiting rooms, and architecture of a healthcare organization (e.g., physician's office, hospital atrium) that reinforce to patients the high quality of care they will experience

independent practice association (IPA): a loose network of physician groups and practices, often formed to increase physicians' negotiating power over HMOs and managed care organizations

integrity: the quality of being whole, sincere, and authentic

intelligence: being knowledgeable about the discipline of marketing and about the products the health marketer is communicating

invisible value: value that a producer builds into its product

justice: ensuring that people are treated fairly to bring about a fair outcome

knowledge: prior experiences and understandings that team members bring to the task at hand and that guide the team's work

licensure: state laws or codes that delineate the scope of practice of specific professions and give qualified professionals who pass a proficiency exam the legal right to practice their trade

long-term care: an array of services, both medical and nonmedical, for people who need help over long periods; often associated with nursing homes

managed care: a prospective reimbursement system designed to control the cost and delivery of healthcare while improving the quality and outcomes of care

market-based economy: a system of production and consumption of goods and services in which transactions and exchanges are based on the rudiments of supply and demand and fundamental competitive principles

market growth: increase in demand for services provided or products sold

market research: efforts to discover and identify the needs of patients, physicians, and the public; may be outsourced or conducted in-house

market strategy: the section of the marketing plan that identifies the target market and what the organization wants to convey so that it reaches the target market effectively and meets the target market's needs

marketing plan: a document that demonstrates how the healthcare organization will implement the already established marketing strategy

Medicaid: a joint state and federal public health insurance program for specific categories of the poor

medical staff privileges: permission to practice in a hospital, granted to physicians who pass the hospital's credentialing process

medical tourism: traveling to other countries to obtain less expensive yet safe, high-quality care

Medicare: a federal public health insurance program primarily for the elderly and for patients with kidney disease

medicine: the profession of healing and caregiving as provided by licensed physicians

Medigap insurance: the informal name for insurance plans sold by private insurance companies to cover healthcare services/products that are not covered by Medicare

message alignment: the synchronization and consistency of a message with the receiver's culture, knowledge, and interests

mission statement: the embodiment and self-image of an organization; a declaration that expresses an organization's highest goals and provides strategic direction

norming: the third, or middle, stage of teamwork; members agree on working styles and processes, conflict decreases, and group cohesiveness develops

objectives: long-term performance and outcome goals

organizational politics: behavior aimed at self-gain, regardless of whether it brings about gain for others

organizational values: standards that govern the behavior of individuals in an organization

organizing: scheduling, team building, delegating, assigning projects and work, and ensuring staff have adequate resources to complete their work

out-of-pocket expenses: non-premium expenses, such as deductibles, that patients must pay for with their own funds

patient: an individual awaiting or under medical care and treatment

patient-centered medical home (PCMH): a healthcare organization designed to provide comprehensive primary care for patients throughout their lives; patients have a "medical home" where healthcare providers, acting on interdisciplinary teams, provide coordinated care so that patients' information is stored at one site

payer mix: the combination of payers, including third parties and individuals, from which a healthcare organization is receiving reimbursement

performing: the fourth stage of teamwork; members engage in and complete the team's work and achieve the team's purpose

physician bonding: ensuring that physicians engage with a hospital closely enough to admit their patients to it exclusively

planning: defining goals and the specific tasks and actions necessary to achieving them

politics: social relations involving authority or power; interests masquerading as a contest of principles or the conduct of public affairs for private advantage

power: the ability to influence someone else to take some action, regardless of whether he or she wants to do so

power by virtue of position: the ability to influence someone else to take some action, regardless of whether he or she wants to do so, derived from the authority awarded to the influencer's position

principal–agent relationship: the principal (patient) gives consent for the agent (caregiver) to have the authority and power to make appropriate decisions on her or his behalf

private health insurers: non-government-owned, for-profit and not-for-profit private businesses that sell health insurance

process conflict: disagreement over workload delegation

profession: a principal calling or vocation based on specialized knowledge that is usually attained through long, intensive academic study

professional code of ethics: ethical/professional standards of conduct/behavior for members of a profession

prospective payment: reimbursement system in which providers know *before* the service is rendered the amount the insurance company will cover

public health: civic activities, laws, and regulations designed to protect the health and well-being of a population

public health insurers: not-for-profit insurance plans owned and run by the federal government or by the states; examples include Medicare, Medicaid, and CHIP

public relations: communicating information about an organization to the public to build understanding and support

relationship conflict: disagreement over personal issues; interpersonal differences

relationship marketing: marketing communications that continuously build on and strengthen the relationships and loyalty among consumers and organizations

retrospective reimbursement: payment system in which the amount the provider is reimbursed is decided by the insurance company after the service has been rendered

return on investment (ROI): a performance measure used to evaluate the success of initiatives that require an investment (in time, effort, and/or money)

risk: uncertainty

situational analysis: an analysis (e.g., a SWOT analysis) of what is happening in an organization's external and internal environments

sliding fee scale: a reimbursement system that uses an individual's income, financial resources, and ability to pay as the basis for determining the amount he or she will pay for a healthcare service

sociability: the ability to build and maintain appropriate and productive professional relationships

social marketing: the creation, communication, and delivery of information, events, programs, and so forth to influence individual behavior for the benefit of not only the individual but also the community and for the common good

stakeholders: people, groups, and organizations that "hold a stake" in an enterprise and are affected by the conduct of people in that enterprise

stigma: a discredited attribute

storming: the second stage of teamwork; as members learn about each other, conflict and emotional issues may arise

strategic planning: design of a plan to achieve agreed-upon goals

strategy: an overarching plan designed to achieve a goal

SWOT analysis: a tool used to identify an organization's internal strengths and weaknesses as well as an organization's external opportunities and threats

tactics: the specific actions taken to achieve a goal

target market: a segment of a population that a provider wants to attract and engage

task conflict: disagreement over the content of decisions relating to a particular task

tax-exempt status of health insurance: the federal provision that treats employer spending on employee health insurance as a tax-deductible business expense, not as taxable income

team-centered: characterized by purposeful exchange, interaction, and collaboration along a spectrum of knowledgeable professionals

third-party payers: the third entity involved in health services transactions, after providers (first) and the patient (second) (A health insurance company is one example of a third-party payer.)

undergraduate medical education: medical school, usually four years in duration

value: relative worth; quality received in exchange for an investment of time, money, or effort

variance: the difference between two items, such as the difference between what was budgeted for a set period and what was actually expensed during that time frame

visible value: value that a customer can see

vision statement: a declaration of an organization's ideal future state, the direction an organization wants to take to get there, and the desired end result

INDEX

ABOUT THE AUTHORS

Leigh W. Cellucci, PhD, is associate professor in the Department of Health Services and Information Management at East Carolina University and a former professor at Francis Marion University and Idaho State University. She was a Fulbright Scholar to India and recipient of a grant for innovative teaching from the American Sociological Association as well as two grants sponsored by the BB&T Leadership Enhancement Fund that focus on leadership development in the classroom. Dr. Cellucci currently serves as editor of the *Journal of Case Studies*, a publication of the Society for Case Research.

Carla Wiggins, PhD, is professor and MHA program director at Weber State University in Ogden, Utah. Dr. Wiggins is a former director of health administration studies at the University of Wisconsin–Milwaukee and former professor and chair of healthcare administration at Idaho State University. She is a prolific author on the topic of health information technology, most recently its role in ambulatory surgery centers.

Tracy J. Farnsworth, EdD, is associate dean and director of the Idaho State University (ISU) Kasiska School of Health Professions in the Division of Health Sciences. Following a distinguished career in hospital and healthcare administration, Dr. Farnsworth joined the ISU Health Care Administration program faculty in 2008. Dr. Farnsworth has written and spoken widely on health system improvement, healthcare reform, and interprofessional education and collaboration.